SELF-ASSESS

MW00986939

Rheumatology

Michael Doherty MD, DMDM, DMDM
Reader and Consultant in Rheumatology
Rheumatology Unit
Nottingham City Hospital
Hucknall Road
Nottingham, UK

Emmanuel George MD, DMDM, DMDM
Arrowe Park Hospital
Upton Road
Upton
Wirral, UK

Ⅳ Mosby-Wolfe

London Baltimore Bogotá Boston Buenos Aires Caracas Carlsbad, CA Chicago Madrid Mexico City Milan Naples, FL
New York Philadelphia St. Louis Sydney Tokyo Toronto Wiesbaden

Project Manager:	Roderick Craig
Developmental Editor:	Deborah Shipman
Production:	Mike Heath
Index:	Jill Halliday
Publisher:	Fiona Foley

Published in 1995 by Mosby-Wolfe, an imprint of Times Mirror International Publishers Limited

Printed by Grafos, S.A. ARTE SOBRE PAPEL

ISBN 0 7234 1968 X

For full details of all Times Mirror International Publishers Limited titles, please write to Times Mirror International Publishers Limited, Lynton House, 7–12 Tavistock Square, London WC1H 9LB, England.

A CIP catalogue record for this book is available from the British Library.

Library of Congress Cataloging-in-Publication Data Applied For

PREFACE

Locomotor symptoms are very common in general practice and hospital-based medicine. Such symptoms may reflect primary rheumatic disease or arise as a manifestation of endocrine, metabolic, or other "general medical" conditions. This book is primarily aimed at trainees in internal medicine and rheumatology but it should also prove of interest to consultant physicians, orthopaedic surgeons and interested general practitioners. If follows a "reader-centred" question and answer format with expansion around key points in each case. We have not attempted a comprehensive coverage of "rheumatology" but have selected a mix of common and unusual locomotor conditions from a wide spectrum of rheumatological and general medical conditions. We have particularly emphasised clinical aspects of the history and examination, and focused on basic investigations, that aid in differential diagnosis. We hope that within each question and answer the reader will find useful information on diagnosis, pathogenesis and management.

ACKNOWLEDGMENTS

We would like to thank the many patients who kindly agreed to be photographed for educational purposes.

Michael Doherty
Emmanuel George

DEDICATION

To Carol, Chris, Mike, Charlie, James, Sally, Emma and Jill

GLOSSARY OF ABBREVIATIONS

AS	ANKYLOSING SPONDYLITIS
CT	CONNECTIVE TISSUE
DIP	DISTAL-INTERPHALANGEAL JOINT
MCPJ	METACARPO-PHALANGEAL JOINT
MCTD	MIXED CONNECTIVE TISSUE DISEASE
MTPJ	METATARSO-PHALANGEAL JOINT
OA	OSTEOARTHRITIS
PIPJ	PROXIMAL-INTERPHALANGEAL JOINT
PsA	PSORIATIC ARTHRITIS
RA	RHEUMATOID ARTHRITIS
RF	RHEUMATOID FACTOR
SLE	SYSTEMIC LUPUS ERYTHEMATOSUS

1 Over a six-month period this fit 26-year-old nurse presented to casualty on three occasions with acute, painful swelling and discolouration of her face, each episode resolving spontaneously over a few weeks. She denied any trauma but on the second occasion her boyfriend was interviewed by Social Services for suspected assault. During the third episode, illustrated here, she also developed synovitis with marked periarticular swelling of her right ankle and midfoot.
(a) What is the diagnosis?
(b) What investigations should be undertaken?

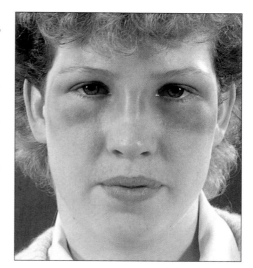

2 A 75-year-old man with RA complained of a painful elbow for three days.
(a) What is the swelling shown?
(b) Does it communicate with the joint?
(c) In what conditions does it commonly become involved?

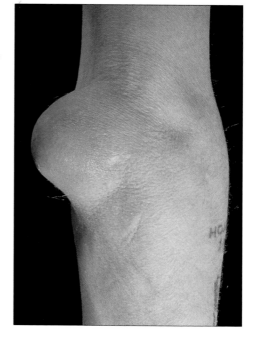

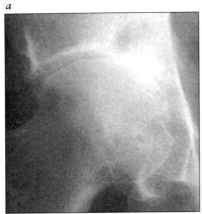

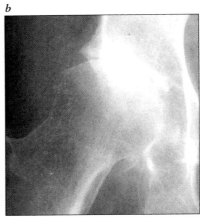

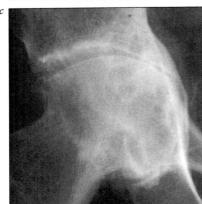

3 These radiographs show different patterns of femoral head migration. (a) What is the underlying condition? (b) Place the patterns in their order of frequency.

4 This 62-year-old woman gave a four-month history of pain around her left groin and upper thigh. The pain was mainly noticeable at night and though initially helped by NSAIDs it had slowly worsened over the last two months and was severely interrupting her sleep. Examination showed normal hip movements.
(a) What features are shown on her radiograph?
(b) What is the diagnosis?

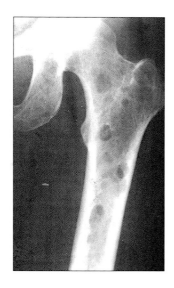

a   *b*

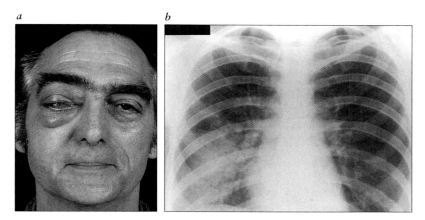

5 This 52-year-old man presented with an eight-week history of a painful right eye, diplopia, and eyelid swelling (Figure *a*). He had recently also suffered several nose bleeds and for three months had noticed a persistent dry cough. He felt generally unwell and had lost weight.
(a) What abnormality is present on his chest radiograph (Figure *b*)?
(b) What is the diagnosis?
(c) What is the treatment?

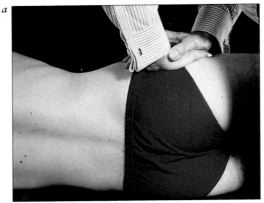

a

6 A previously fit 30-year-old man presented with a six-week history of progressive pain affecting his left buttock and posterior thigh, which was worse on weight-bearing but also present at night. Lumbar spine and hip examination was normal and there were no neurological signs. Standing on his left leg alone, and stressing his sacroiliac joint (Figure *a*), both reproduced his pain.

(a) What abnormalities are present on his pelvis radiograph (Figure *b*) and CT scan (Figure *c*)?

(b) What is the diagnosis?

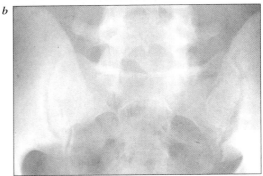

b

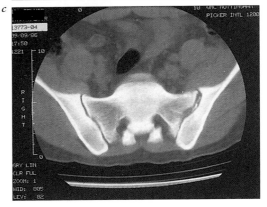

c

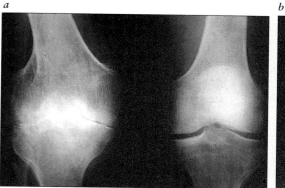
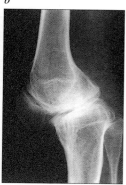

7 This 40-year-old man had suffered recurrent attacks of pain and swelling in both his elbows, his right knee and both ankles since the age of seven. Symptoms had become chronic at these sites over the previous 15 years.
(a) What abnormalities are shown on his AP (Figure *a*) and lateral (Figure *b*) knee radiographs?
(b) What is the diagnosis?

8 (a) Describe the abnormalities on this lateral cervical spine x-ray.
(b) What is the likely underlying disease process?
(c) What is the association between cervical spine and peripheral joint involvement in this disease?

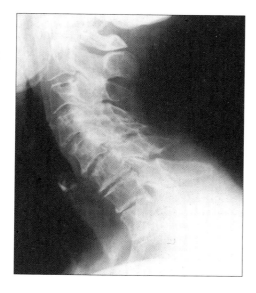

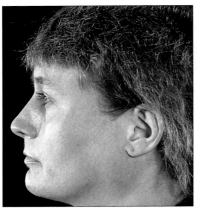

9 A 45-year-old woman complained of frequent cracking of her lips and fissuring of her tongue. She was otherwise well but was currently under investigation for dyspareunia. A simple eye test confirmed the clinical diagnosis.
(a) What abnormality is apparent in the photograph?
(b) What was the eye test?
(c) What is the likely diagnosis?

a

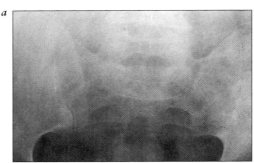

b

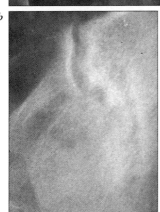

10 A 24-year-old man gave a ten-week history of non-progressive "sciatica" affecting his left buttock and thigh, and right inferior heel pain. One year before he had suffered self-limiting right ankle and left knee synovitis. He gave no history of skin, eye or bowel problems. The only sign on examination was tenderness over his right plantar fascia origin.
(a) What abnormalities are seen on his pelvis radiograph (Figure *a*) and the close-up (Figure *b*)?
(b) What is the likely diagnosis?

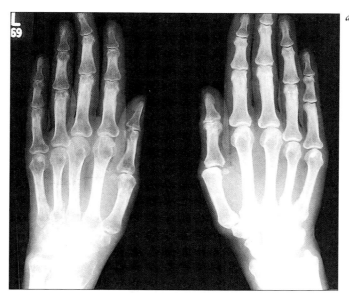

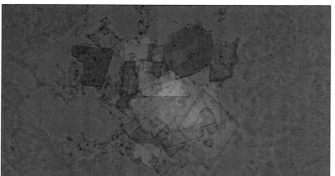

11 This 38-year-old Asian woman gave an eight-month history of progressive pain and stiffness of her left wrist. Her husband, a GP, had tried NSAIDs and physiotherapy (for presumptive extensor tenosynovitis) without success. Examination revealed mild swelling over the dorsum of her wrist and restricted wrist movement with stress pain; there was generalised tenderness, maximal over the ulnar aspect of her carpus.

(a) What abnormalities are present on her hand radiograph (Figure *a*)?

(b) What is shown in the aspirate from her wrist (Figure *b*; compensated polarised light microscopy ×200)?

(c) What is the likely diagnosis?

11

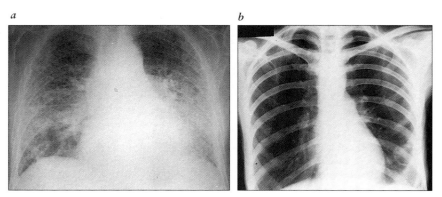

12 Figures *a* and *b* are radiographs belonging to two patients with RA.
(a) What do they show?
(b) What other pulmonary manifestations occur in RA?

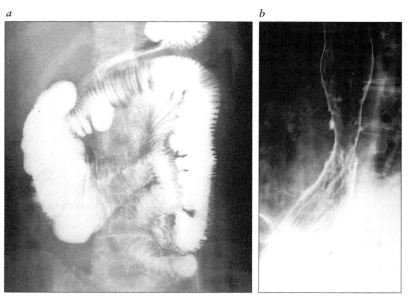

13 Figures *a* and *b* are barium contrast studies undertaken on two patients with the same connective tissue disease.
(a) What abnormalities are present in each?
(b) What is the likely underlying connective tissue disease?

14 This 55-year-old woman has had seropositive nodular RA for 20 years. She has no eye discomfort or visual disturbance.
(a) What eye abnormalities are present?
(b) What is the diagnosis?

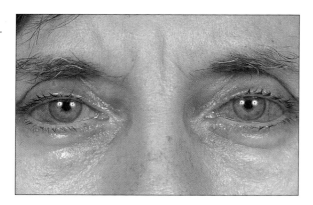

15 This 53-year-old man presented with bilateral knee pain. Knee examination (Figure *a*) revealed marked crepitus, bony swelling but normal range of movement.
(a) What abnormalities are present on his standing knee radiograph (Figure *b*)?
(b) What is the diagnosis?

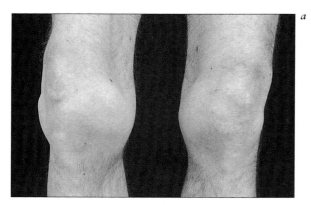

a

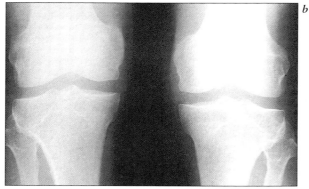

b

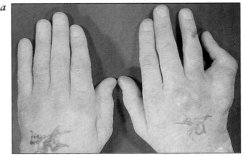

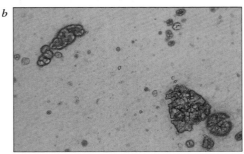

16 A 47-year-old alcoholic labourer was admitted with confusion, hypotension and dehydration. Over the previous three months he had noticed pain and swelling affecting his wrists, metacarpophalangeal joints, elbows, knees and feet. He was resuscitated and treated initially as septicaemia. Examination revealed synovitis of symptomatic joints, damage and subluxation to several small joints and large fluctuant periarticular swellings over extensor surfaces of elbows, knees, and hands (Figure *a*). Aspiration of joints and swellings revealed turbid fluid, sterile on culture, containing lipid-staining material (Figure *b*).
(a) What radiographic abnormalities are present in Figure *c*?
(b) What is the diagnosis?

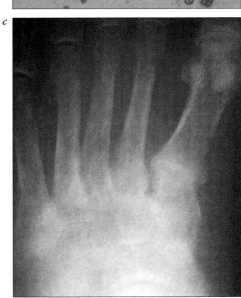

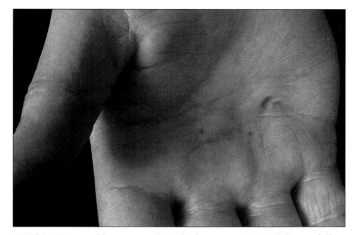

17 This 67-year-old man complained of a progressive inability to fully extend several fingers of his left hand.
(a) What is the diagnosis?
(b) Which fingers are most commonly affected?
(c) What are the aetiological associations?

a

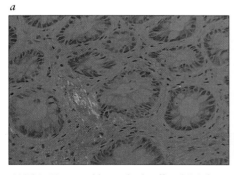

b

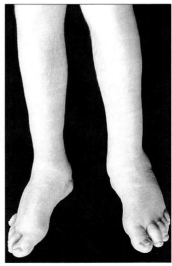

18 This 59-year-old man had suffered RA for 18 years. Over the previous six weeks he had noticed persistent lower leg and ankle swelling (Figure *b*), which was resistant to tight support stockings. Subsequent investigations, including proteinuria (8gm/24 hours), led to a tissue biopsy (Figure *a*).
(a) What tissue (×100) is shown in the biopsy?
(b) What is the diagnosis?

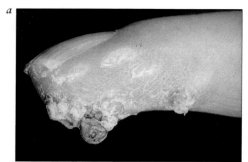

19 This 55-year-old woman gave a long history of Raynaud's phenomenon and progressive stiffening of both hands with occasional distal ulceration and discharge (Figure *a*). She was receiving antacids for troublesome heartburn but was otherwise well.
(a) What does her hand radiograph (Figure *b*) show?
(b) What is the likely diagnosis?

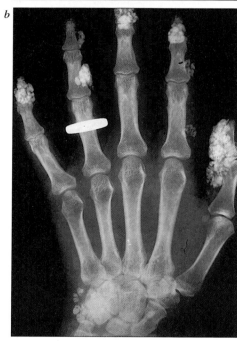

20 This 38-year-old man, who had been on haemodialysis for five years and had undergone two failed renal transplants, developed chronic pain, stiffness and swelling in several interphalangeal joints (Figure *a*) with superimposed self-limiting attacks of acute synovitis, each lasting from one to three weeks.

(a) What changes are shown on his hand radiograph (Figure *b*)?

(b) What is shown in the synovial fluid (compensated polarised light microscopy ×400; Figure *c*) aspirated from an affected interphalangeal joint?

(c) What is the diagnosis?

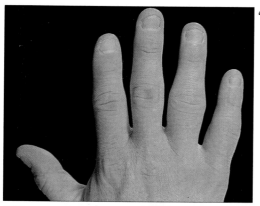

a

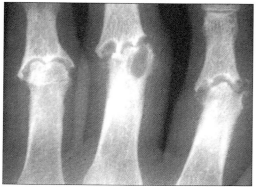

b

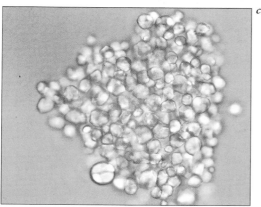

c

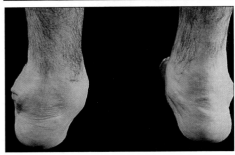

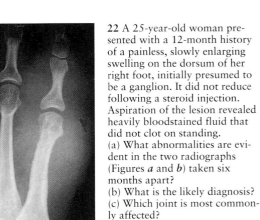

21 This 43-year-old man has longstanding RA.
(a) Describe his foot abnormalities in Figures *a* and *b*.
(b) Which tendon is mainly affected in the hindfoot deformity? What are its insertions and functions?

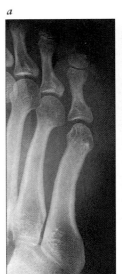 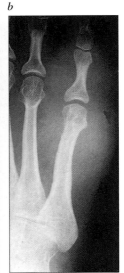

22 A 25-year-old woman presented with a 12-month history of a painless, slowly enlarging swelling on the dorsum of her right foot, initially presumed to be a ganglion. It did not reduce following a steroid injection. Aspiration of the lesion revealed heavily bloodstained fluid that did not clot on standing.
(a) What abnormalities are evident in the two radiographs (Figures *a* and *b*) taken six months apart?
(b) What is the likely diagnosis?
(c) Which joint is most commonly affected?

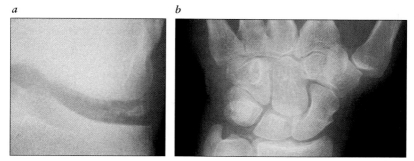

a   b

23 This 38-year-old woman had suffered eight acute, self-limiting attacks of pain and
swelling (with erythema) affecting her knees and left wrist over the previous ten
years. She was otherwise well and there was no family history of joint disease. Full
locomotor and general examination was unremarkable.
(a) What abnormality is present on her knee (Figure *a*) and wrist (Figure *b*) radiographs?
(b) What investigations would you undertake?

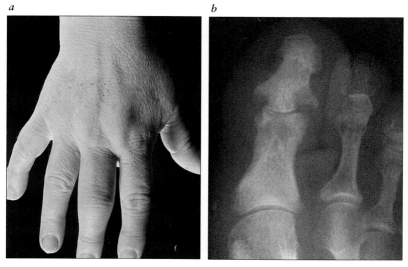

a   b

24 A fit 37-year-old man presented with a swollen and painful right middle finger
with inability to fully flex. He had similar involvement of his right big toe.
(a) What term describes the clinical appearance in Figure *a*?
(b) What abnormalities are present in the x-ray of his right big toe (Figure *b*)?
(c) What is the likely diagnosis?

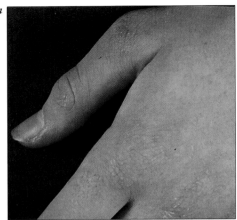

a

25 A 57-year-old woman presented with a four-week history of increasing lethargy and weakness, with difficulty climbing stairs or rising from a low seat. Examination confirmed trunk, neck and shoulder girdle weakness as well as a rash (Figure *a*). For two months she had also noticed irregular bowel habits; her barium enema is shown in Figure *b*.

(a) What is the most likely diagnosis?

(b) What muscle investigations are appropriate?

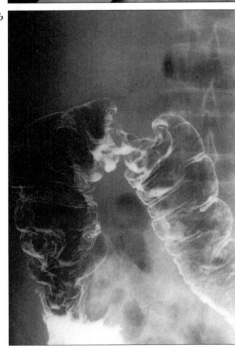

b

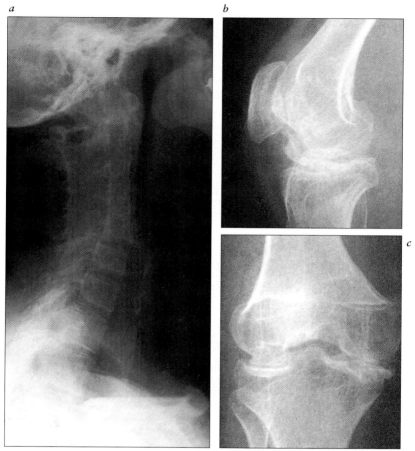

a

b

c

26 A 19-year-old boy presented with a six-month history of progressive knee pain. At age eight he had developed inflammatory polyarthritis that required frequent hospital visits, but since age 12 he had been well. Current examination revealed reduced movement, bony enlargement and crepitus (but no inflammation) of both his knees, wrists and several small hand joints; lateral cervical flexion was also restricted.

(a) What abnormalities are present on the cervical spine (Figure *a*) and knee (Figures *b* and *c*) x-rays?

(b) What is the diagnosis?

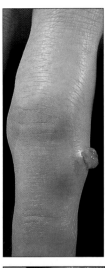

27 This 46-year-old woman presented with an 18-month history of pain and stiffness sequentially affecting several DIPJs and PIPJs. Her left middle finger was the most symptomatic and showed normal movement with stress pain, and posterolateral swelling. Puncture of the swelling released gelatinous material.
(a) What is the material?
(b) What is the diagnosis?

a
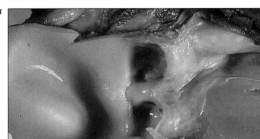

28 These two figures illustrate manifestations of SLE. What are the lesions in each figure called?

b
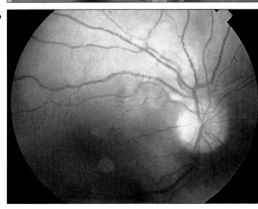

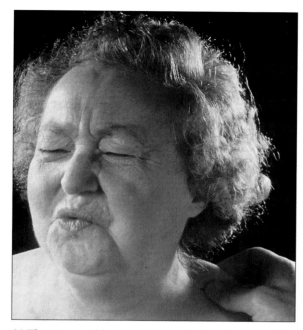

29 This 60-year-old woman presented with a three-year history of severe neck and back pain, marked fatiguability, and intermittent abdominal pain and headaches. She had also noticed generalised early morning stiffness and swelling of both hands. She had had to give up her part-time secretarial job because of pain, tiredness, and increasing forgetfulness. Examination showed marked tenderness on skin-fold rolling over trapezius (illustrated) and on palpation at several muscle and enthesis sites. The locomotor and general examination was otherwise unremarkable.

(a) What is the likely diagnosis?

(b) What investigations would you undertake?

a

b

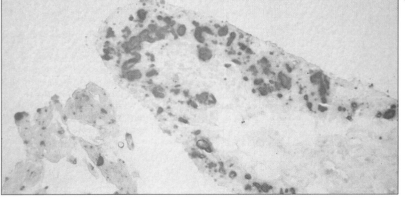

c

30 This fit 78-year-old woman developed rapidly progressive pain in her right hip and after just 12 months came for hip replacement (full blood count and ESR were normal). One year later she developed severe pain in her right knee. Examination revealed a large cool effusion, lateral compartment tenderness and instability. Her symptoms progressed and she again required total joint replacement.
(a) What is the differential diagnosis of her pre-operative hip (Figure *a*) and knee (Figure *b*) radiographs?
(b) What is demonstrated in her knee synovium (Figure *c*; alizarin red stain ×200)?
(c) What is the diagnosis?

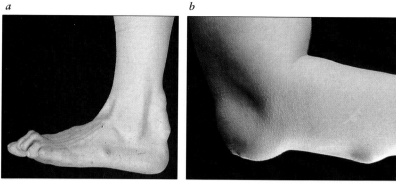

a   *b*

31 Figures *a* and *b* are of the same patient with rheumatoid arthritis.
(a) Describe the principal abnormalities in Figure *a*.
(b) What are the abnormalities in Figure *b* and how can you differentiate them?
(c) What would histology of the firm swellings reveal?

32 A 27-year-old man presented with a three-week history of frequent bloody diarrhoea and weight loss. He had no history of joint symptoms other than intermittent mild left buttock ache. Examination revealed no skin or locomotor abnormality.
(a) What abnormalities are evident in his plain abdominal radiograph?
(b) What are the probable diagnoses?

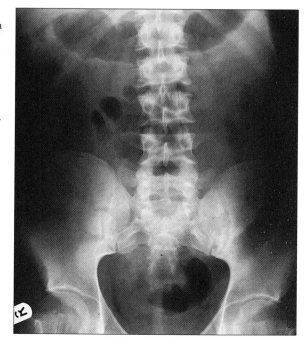

a
b

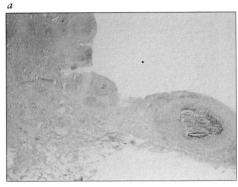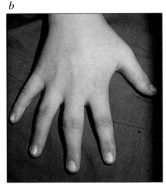

33 Six weeks before presentation this 13-year-old girl had developed an acutely painful, red, swollen right middle finger. It initially settled on ten days of flucloxacillin from her GP but two weeks later slowly recurred. She denied any prior trauma and was otherwise well. Examination revealed synovitis of the middle finger PIPJ (Figure *b*). A plain radiograph showed only soft tissue swelling. Histology of removed synovium is in Figure *a*.
What is the diagnosis?

34 A 56-year-old Asian woman with long-standing epilepsy presented with a six-month history of progressive weakness, with particular difficulty climbing stairs. She also complained of pains around both hips, which was worse on weight-bearing.
(a) What abnormality is present on her left hip x-ray?
(b) What is the likely diagnosis?
(c) What are the likely causes in this patient?

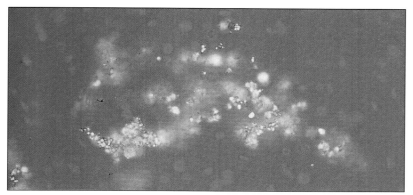

35 A 67-year-old woman suffered an exacerbation of her longstanding right knee OA and received an intra-articular steroid injection from her GP. The next day her knee was much more painful and inflamed, she felt feverish and developed uncomfortable facial flushing. Both knees showed signs of OA (crepitus, restricted movement, mild varus deformity) with a moderate, warm effusion and joint-line tenderness on the right. Her knee was aspirated; the Gram stain was normal and subsequent culture proved negative. Her flushing and feverishness had resolved 48 hours later.
(a) What is present in her knee fluid (compensated polarised light microscopy ×400) shown here?
(b) What is the diagnosis?

36 A 12-year-old boy presented with acute knee and ankle pain, then rapidly developed an extensive rash over his legs and buttocks. He gave a history of a viral illness ten days earlier.
(a) What is the likely diagnosis?
(b) What musculoskeletal signs and symptoms are usually associated with this condition?

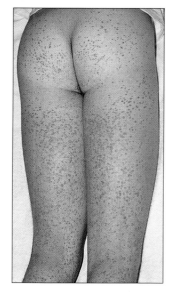

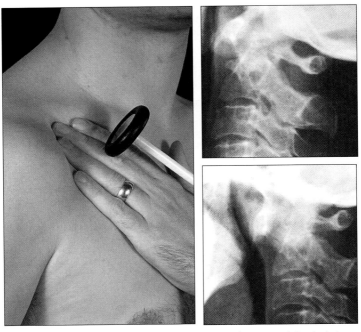

37 This 54-year-old man with a 20-year history of RA complained of clumsiness and worsening hand function over the three months prior to referral. He had also noticed unusual difficulty in moving around the house and getting in and out of his car. Both pectoralis jerks (Figure *a*) were brisk but his jaw jerk was normal (not brisk).
(a) What can you deduce from his pectoralis and jaw jerks?
(b) What is shown on his lateral cervical spine extension (Figure *b*) and flexion (Figure *c*) radiographs?
(c) What is the likely cause of his altered function?

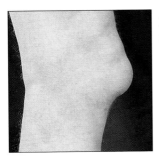

38 A 36-year-old bricklayer presented with a six-week history of painful swelling of his anterior right knee. He had no other symptoms.
(a) What is the diagnosis?
(b) What is the treatment?

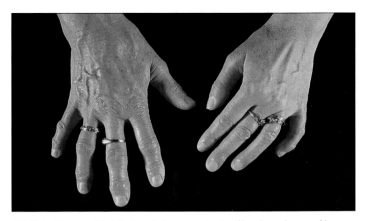

39 This 67-year-old right-handed woman had suffered weakness of her left hand following a childhood illness. In her 40s she developed, over several years, pain, stiffness and swelling of the interphalangeal joints in her right hand. Her symptoms slowly settled and had resolved once she was in her 50s. At 67 she was now being referred with bilateral knee pain. Her left hand showed global weakness, with weakness of forearm flexors and extensors; sensation was normal.
(a) What rheumatic condition affects her right hand?
(b) What abnormalities are apparent in her left hand?
(c) Explain the discordance between her hands.

40 This is the foot radiograph of a 34-year-old woman with a two-year history of inflammatory polyarthritis.
(a) What abnormalities are present?
(b) What is the diagnosis?

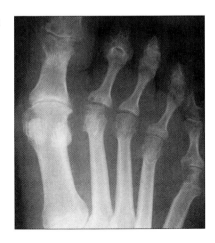

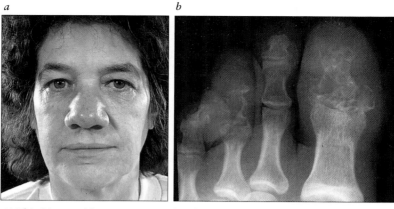

41 This 54-year-old woman presented with a two-year history of pain and swelling of her left knee and several toes. She felt generally unwell, had lost weight and had noticed tender, red swelling of her nose and face (Figure *a*).
(a) What is her facial lesion?
(b) What abnormalities are present on her foot radiograph (Figure *b*)?
(c) What is the diagnosis?

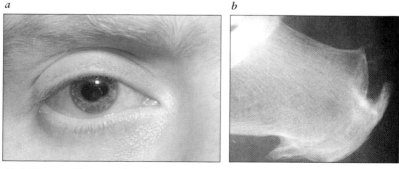

42 A 27-year-old man with a chronic inflammatory eye condition complained of persistent heel pain and a chronic left knee monoarthritis. He gave no history of skin disease.
(a) What is his eye problem (Figure *a*)?
(b) What abnormalities are present on his heel x-ray (Figure *b*)?
(c) What is the likely diagnosis?

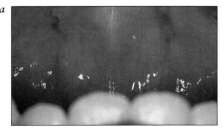

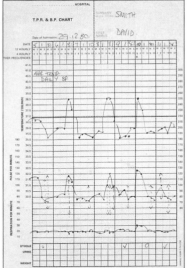

43 A five-year-old boy was admitted with a four-week history of feeling unwell, night sweats, arthralgia, sore throat, loss of appetite and weight loss. A faint erythematous macular rash had been noticed on his trunk by his mother. Examination revealed symmetrical synovitis of the wrists, MCPJs, ankles and knees with painful restriction of neck movement; no rash was evident.
(a) What abnormalities are observed in Figure *a*?
(b) Describe his temperature chart (Figure *b*).
(c) What is the likely diagnosis?

44 A previously fit 76-year-old man presented with a three-month history of progressive low back pain that had started three weeks after successful transurethral prostatectomy. He had also noted weakness and parasthesia of both legs. The pain was now so severe that he was limited to crawling around the floor on all fours.
(a) What investigation and abnormalities are shown in this x-ray?
(b) What is the likely diagnosis?

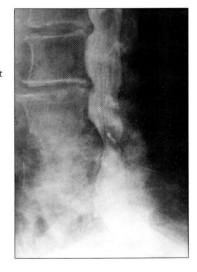

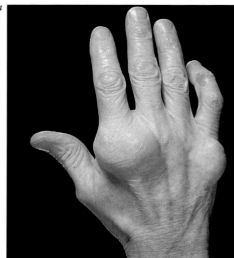

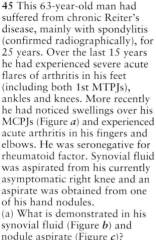

45 This 63-year-old man had suffered from chronic Reiter's disease, mainly with spondylitis (confirmed radiographically), for 25 years. Over the last 15 years he had experienced severe acute flares of arthritis in his feet (including both 1st MTPJs), ankles and knees. More recently he had noticed swellings over his MCPJs (Figure *a*) and experienced acute arthritis in his fingers and elbows. He was seronegative for rheumatoid factor. Synovial fluid was aspirated from his currently asymptomatic right knee and an aspirate was obtained from one of his hand nodules.

(a) What is demonstrated in his synovial fluid (Figure *b*) and nodule aspirate (Figure *c*)?

(b) What is the diagnosis of his locomotor problems?

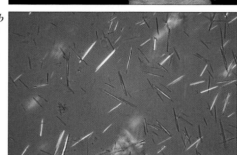

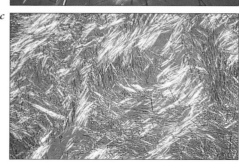

46 This 43-year-old patient had an 18-history of polyarthritis, resulting in hand and feet deformities. She was rheumatoid factor positive and had been told that she had rheumatoid arthritis. She also described Raynaud's phenomenon and photosensitivity. She was now referred because of the report on a recent hand x-ray, shown here.
(a) What abnormalities are present on the x-ray?
(b) What is the likely cause of her arthropathy?

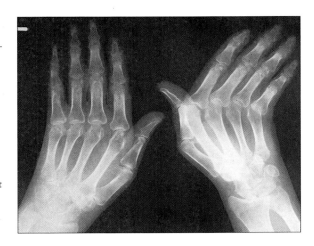

47 (a) What abnormality is evident in this patient with RA?
(b) What complications may result?
(c) What other conditions may cause this?

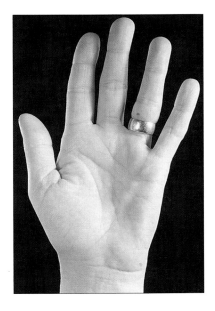

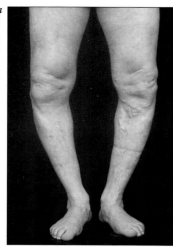

48 This 64-year-old man gave an eight-year history of pain, stiffness and intermittent swelling affecting both knees. Examination revealed modest effusions, crepitus, medial joint-line tenderness, and bilateral varus (Figure *a*). His lying and standing left AP knee films are shown in Figure *b*.
(a) What is the diagnosis?
(b) What factors may relate to its progression?

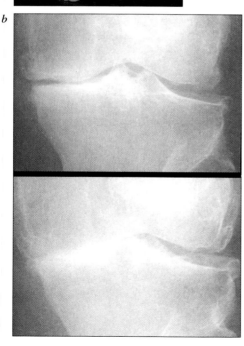

49 This 62-year-old woman had a three-year history of bilateral, symmetrical polyarthritis affecting small joints of her hands, feet, knees and elbows. She had been diagnosed as RA. She then developed small, purplish nodules around her nailfolds, fingers (Figure *a*), nose and elbows. She was persistently seronegative for rheumatoid factor.

(a) What abnormalities are shown on her hand radiograph (Figure *b*)?

(b) What is the diagnosis?

(c) How is it confirmed?

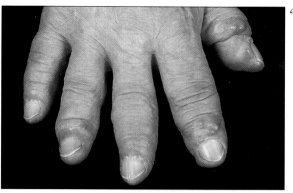

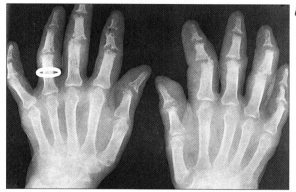

50 (a) Describe the abnormalities in this 70-year-old woman with long-standing arthritis.

(b) What is the likely underlying disease?

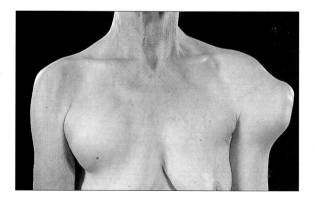

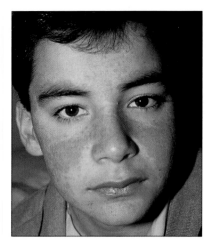

51 This 17-year-old boy presented with a facial rash, generalised fatigue and arthralgia of his hands, knees and feet for five weeks. Examination revealed extensor tenosynovitis of the hands and hard palate ulceration. Urine testing revealed protein-uria with casts on microscopy.
(a) What is the likely diagnosis?
(b) What treatment is he likely to require?

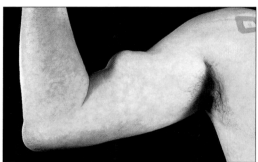

52 This otherwise fit 53-year-old car mechanic developed pain around his right upper humerus. His GP diagnosed bicipital ten-dinitis and gave him a local injection. His pain wors-ened and he was referred urgently to hospital.
What is the diagnosis, obvi-ous on inspection?

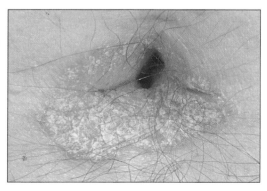

53 A 27-year-old man with unexplained knee synovitis was referred by the ortho-paedic surgeons. Careful examination revealed the finding shown here.
(a) What is the likely cause of this skin lesion?
(b) What are its mucocuta-neous features and what other concealed sites should be examined?
(c) What are the associa-tions with arthropathy?

54 This 76-year-old woman had suffered pain and stiffness in both knees for ten years. Three days after hospitalisation for acute myocardial infarction (complicated by complete heart block that required temporary pacing and diuretics) she developed severe, painful swelling of her right knee. Aspiration revealed uniformly blood-stained fluid (Figure *a*).
(a) What is evident on synovial fluid microscopy (Figure *b*; ×400)?
(b) What is the likely diagnosis?

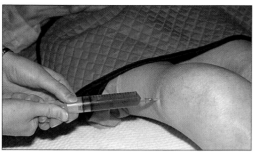

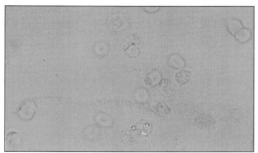

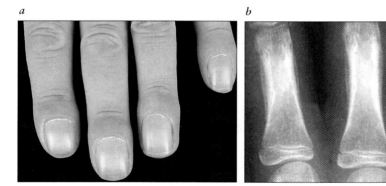

55 This 22-year-old man with known cystic fibrosis (predominant lung involvement) gave a one-year history of painful wrists, metacarpophalangeal joints, elbows and ankles. Elevation of affected limbs relieved his pain. Examination revealed tenderness of affected joints, distal forearms and humeri, and mild synovitis with restricted movement of knees and wrists. His fingers are shown in Figure *a*.
(a) What change is present on his hand radiograph (Figure *b*)?
(b) What is the locomotor diagnosis?

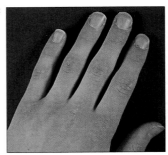 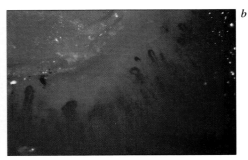

56 This 15-year-old boy presented with a four-week history of weakness, weight loss, painful wrists, metacarpophalangeal and proximal interphalangeal joints, and a rash. The rash affected the back of both hands (Figure *a*) and both elbows, and he had mild synovitis of his symptomatic joints. He had symmetrical weakness and tenderness of his proximal girdle muscles.
(a) What nailfold abnormality is demonstrated in Figure *b*?
(b) What is the diagnosis?

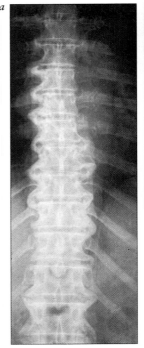 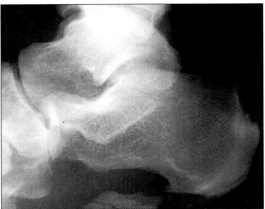

57 This 56-year-old businessman presented with pain under his left heel that was worse on weight bearing. He had no other symptoms. Examination revealed localised tenderness around his plantar fascia insertion, but there was also restricted thoracic expansion and lumbar spine anterior and lateral flexion. His thoracic spine (Figure *a*) and lateral heel (Figure *b*) radiographs are shown.
(a) What is the diagnosis?
(b) What are the associations?

58 This 36-year-old carpenter complained of pain over the lateral aspect of his elbow that was worse when using a screwdriver. His pain (site indicated by hatching) was provoked by holding a full kettle with his hand above but not below (Figure *a*) the handle. Resisted active wrist extension (Figure *b*) reproduced his pain. What is the diagnosis?

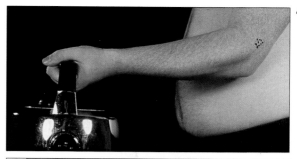

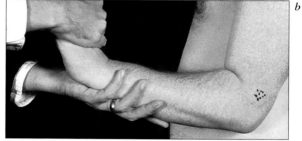

59 (a) Describe the abnormalities on this hand radiograph.
(b) What is the most likely diagnosis?
(c) Which arthropathies commonly result in bony ankylosis?

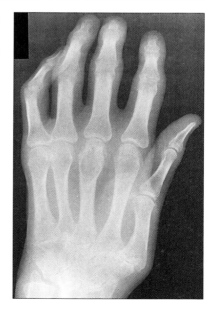

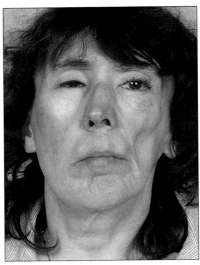 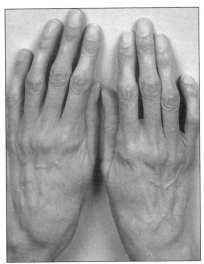

60 This 47-year-old woman gave a long history of severe backpain and arthralgia of the knees, shoulders, hindfoot and wrists. She had also suffered recurrent eye problems. Examination revealed marked kyphoscoliosis in addition to the features evident in Figures *a* and *b* above. Several first-degree relatives suffered similar eye and joint problems.
(a) What is her underlying condition?
(b) What is the basic defect?

61 A 67-year-old overweight woman had presented to her GP six weeks prior to referral complaining of severe left knee pain localised to the medial aspect. This had started suddenly with no preceding trauma. The pain was continuous, particularly bad at night and aggravated by weight-bearing. It was improved by NSAIDs and rest. At referral she had tenderness over the medial anterior femoral condyle and a small effusion.
(a) What is evident on her knee x-ray?
(b) What is the diagnosis?

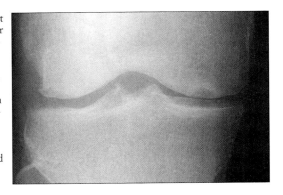

62 A 67-year-old woman presented a two-week history of painful hand discoloration (Figure *a*). She described Raynaud's phenomenon for the past three years and had noticed tightness of her fingers, increasing difficulties with her dentures due to problems opening her mouth (Figure *b*), and difficulty fully closing her eyes (Figure *c*). Doppler examination confirmed all pulses were present and normal. Biochemistry and blood tests were normal except for a positive ANA and anti-centromere antibodies.

(a) Describe the abnormalities seen in the Figures *a*, *b* and *c*.

(b) What is the diagnosis and what complication has occurred?

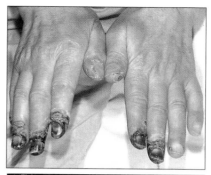
a

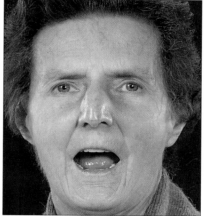
b

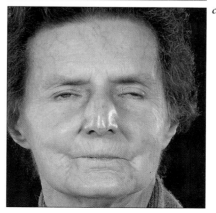
c

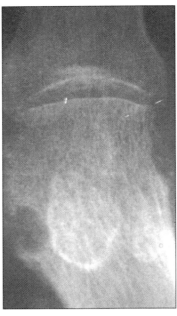

63 A thin 45-year-old male taxi driver gave a 20-year history of recurrent acute attacks of severe pain and swelling affecting his feet, ankles and knees. He had previously suffered 3 episodes of renal colic with no cause found. He drank only moderate amounts of alcohol and was on no regular medication.
(a) What abnormality is shown on his right 1st MTPJ radiograph?
(b) What is the likely diagnosis?
(c) What investigations would you undertake?

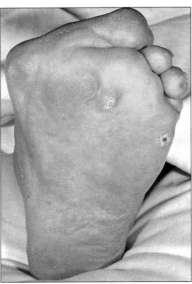

64 These are the feet of a woman with a 12-year history of RA.
Describe the abnormalities.

65 A 68-year-old woman presented with intermittent pain and stiffness affecting several DIPJs and her left hip. Examination revealed painful limitation of left hip internal rotation. What three conditions are discernible on her hip (Figure *a*) and hand (Figure *b*) x-rays?

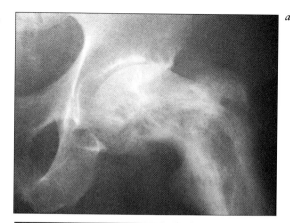

a

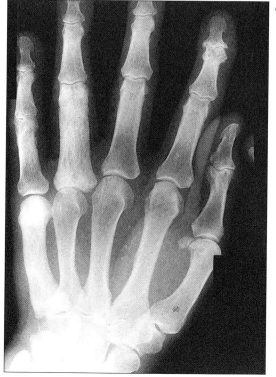

b

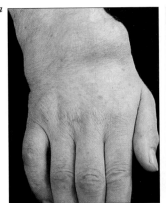
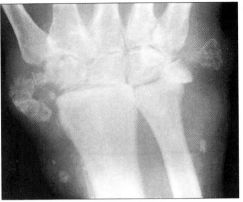

66 This 50-year-old man had developed an acutely painful, swollen right wrist that was unassociated with preceding trauma two years before. The wrist swelling (Figure *a*) had persisted with little discomfort, but he had noticed progressive difficulties with right hand function, which was the reason for referral.
(a) What abnormalities are present on his wrist radiograph (Figure *b*)?
(b) What is the diagnosis?

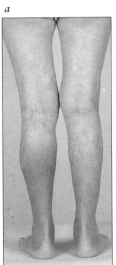
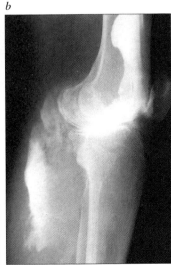

67 This 54-year-old woman with a 10-year history of RA developed acute pain and swelling in her left calf (Figure *a*). She was admitted to a medical ward and commenced heparin. Venography was technically difficult and the result inconclusive. Her pain worsened dramatically after 12 hours so a further investigation was undertaken (Figure *b*).

(a) What abnormality is shown as a result?
(b) How would you manage this patient?

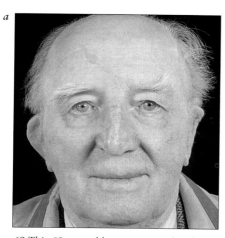

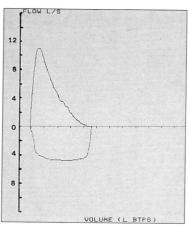

68 This 60-year-old man presented with an 18-month history of intermittent mild synovitis of the wrists and knees. He had also noticed intermittent ear discomfort and tenderness. All previous investigations had been normal apart from a raised ESR.
(a) What signs are evident in Figure *a*?
(b) What abnormality is demonstrated in his flow loop (Figure *b*)?
(c) What is the diagnosis?

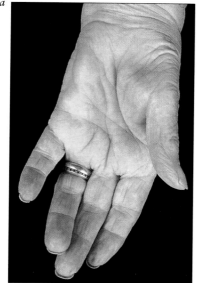

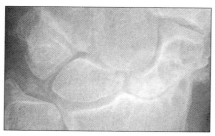

69 This 70-year-old woman gave a four-month history of numbness affecting her left thumb, index and middle finger. This was most noticeable when she awoke in the mornings and was accompanied by aching in the flexor aspect of her forearm. For several years she had suffered intermittent pain in both knees and left wrist. Examination revealed mild synovitis of her left wrist and localised wasting (Figure *a*).
(a) What changes are present in her wrist radiograph (Figure *b*)?
(b) What is the likely diagnosis?

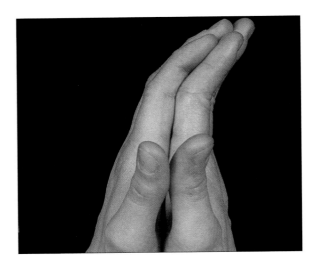

70 This fit 17-year-old ballet dancer was referred with back pain. Previous blood tests and x-rays had been normal but this photograph demonstrates a particular clinical finding.
(a) What is the diagnosis ?
(b) What associated abnormalities would you look for?

a   *b*

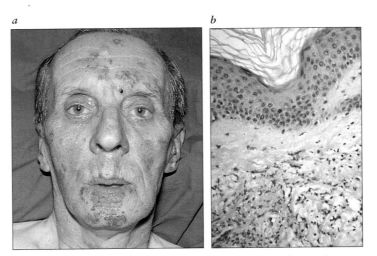

71 This 65-year-old man presented with a six-day history of extensive facial rash (Figure *a*). Over the previous three weeks he had noticed similar lesions on his arms and legs, with arthralgia of elbows, knees and ankles.
(a) What features are evident in the histology of a biopsed lesion (Figure *b*)?
(b) What is the diagnosis?

72 This 46-year-old man complained of low back pain for three years. He gave a history of back problems as a child, which had required three months in hospital in a plaster cast.
(a) What abnormalities are shown on his x-ray?
(b) What condition did he have as a child?

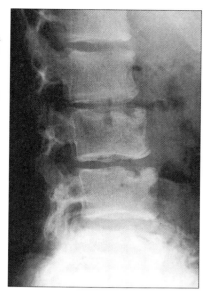

a   *b*

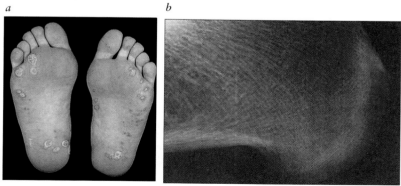

73 A young merchant seaman presented with a two-week history of persistent bilateral heel pain that was worse on walking, and acute synovitis of his left knee, both ankles and right third toe.
(a) What are the skin lesions on his soles (Figure *a*)?
(b) What abnormality is present on his heel x-ray (Figure *b*)?
(c) What is the diagnosis?

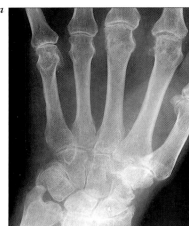

a

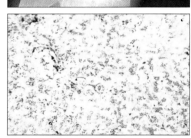

b

74 This 48-year-old solicitor presented with a three-year history of pain and stiffness affecting his hips, ankles, wrists and MCPJs. Examination showed crepitus and restricted movement of affected joints with no overt synovitis. General examination was unremarkable.
(a) What changes are present on his hand radiograph (Figure *a*)?
(b) What tissue was subsequently biopsied (Figure *b*) and what does it show?
(c) What is the diagnosis?

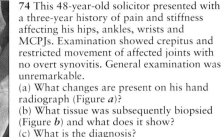

a   *b*

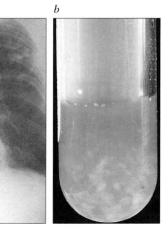

75 This chest radiograph is of a 57-year-old woman with long-standing active RA. Fluid obtained by chest aspiration is shown alongside.
(a) What does the chest x-ray show (Figure *a*)?
(b) What are the particles in the aspirated fluid (Figure *b*) usually called and where are they more usually found?
(c) What is their composition?

76 This 53-year-old woman with insulin-dependent diabetes developed acute pain and swelling over the dorsum of her right foot, with flattening of the longitudinal and transverse arches. Figure *a* and the radiograph in Figure *b* were taken three months later.
What is the diagnosis?

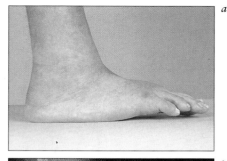

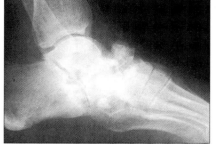

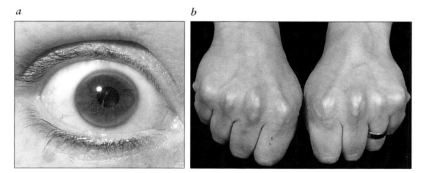

77 This 27-year-old woman complained of recurrent, short-lived episodes of painful knee swelling over the previous four years. She was a keen runner and had experienced four episodes of Achilles tendinitis. Examination was normal apart from the two signs illustrated.
(a) What lesions are present in her eye (Figure *a*) and hands (Figure *b*)?
(b) What is the diagnosis?
(c) What is the important association?

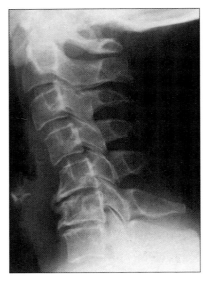

78 For three years this 59-year-old woman had complained of intermittent pain and stiffness affecting the back of her neck with radiation down to both shoulders that was worse on neck movements and when carrying shopping. For six months she had noted paraesthesia affecting the back of her right forearm, thumb and index finger; this was relieved by sitting on her sofa and resting her abducted arm over its side. More recently, however, she complained of right hand clumsiness and numbness (thumb, index, middle finger) that occurred for one hour after waking up. Examination revealed diminished pin-prick sensation over her right thumb and index finger and reduced biceps and supinator jerks. There was no weakness. Tinel's and Phalen's tests reproduced paraesthesia and numbness in her hand.
(a) What changes are apparent on her lateral neck radiograph?
(b) What is the likely diagnosis?

a

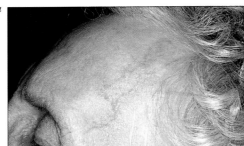

b

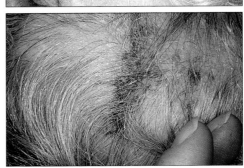

79 A 77-year-old woman gave a one-month history of malaise and fatigue. Two weeks earlier she had developed painful scalp lesions diagnosed by her GP as zoster. Two days before this picture was taken she developed severe bitemporal headache. She presented to casualty with ocular pain, diplopia and photophobia. Fundoscopy revealed pallor and oedema of the disc with several small exudates and haemorrhages.
(a) Describe the features shown in Figures *a* and *b*.
(b) What is the diagnosis?
(c) What treatment would you give immediately?

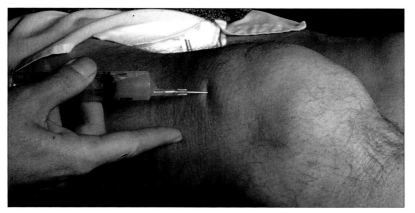

80 This 55-year-old technician developed acute severe pain and swelling of his right knee and felt generally unwell. Over the previous week he had experienced an exacerbation of his long-standing asthma; this was now improving with adjustment of inhalers. Over the previous ten years he had suffered acute episodes of painful swelling in his feet, diagnosed by his GP as gout, but had never had knee problems. On examination he had a fever (38.5°C) and a hot, tense knee effusion. The knee radiograph undertaken in casualty was normal apart from showing an effusion and soft tissue swelling. Aspiration revealed turbid fluid (above).
(a) What is the principal differential diagnosis?
(b) What investigations might be helpful in the acute stage?
(c) What drug therapy would you institute?

81 (a) Describe the abnormalities present in this patient with RA.
(b) List other characteristic finger and thumb deformities found in RA.

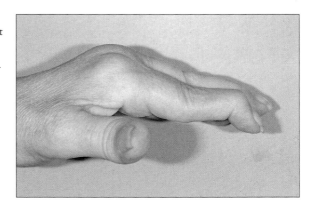

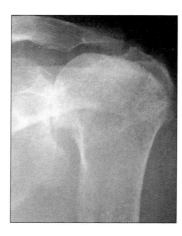

82 This is the x-ray of a 65-year-old man with a chronic history of pain and limited movement of the left shoulder.
(a) What does the x-ray show?
(b) What is the most likely underlying pathology?
(c) What is the function and composition of this anatomical structure?

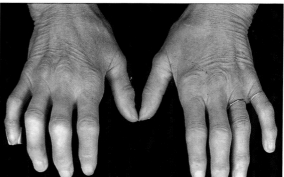

83 A 57-year-old woman complained of progressively stiff, cold hands and arthralgia of her wrists, MCPJs and knees.
(a) What skin changes are evident in the photograph?
(b) What is the likely diagnosis?

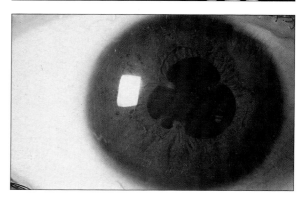

84 This is the dilated pupil of a seven-year-old girl with a two-year history of oligoarthritis.
(a) What abnomality is present?
(b) What is the likely primary diagnosis?
(c) What antibody associates with this eye complication?

85 A 78-year-old man presented with increasing central low back pain. Examination revealed loss of lumbar lordosis and reduced, painful extension. Other movements showed mild restriction.
(a) What abnormalities are present on his lateral radiograph?
(b) What is the likely cause of his symptoms?

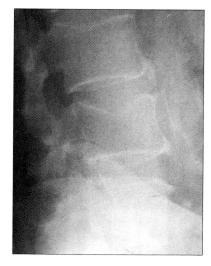

86 A 47-year-old man with chronic renal failure on long-term haemodialysis complained of increasing hand pain and ill-defined widespread aches.
(a) What abnormalities are demonstrated on his hand radiograph (middle finger)?
(b) What is the underlying biochemical abnormality?

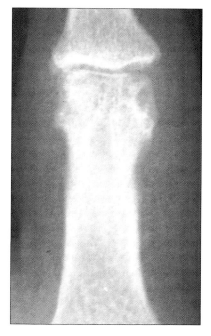

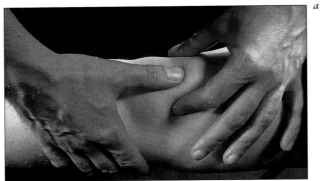

87 This 55-year-old woman presented with intermittent right anterior knee pain. She could walk well on the flat but her pain was most noticeable going up and down stairs and down the hill from her house. Stressing her patello-femoral joint ("patellar grind" – Figure *a*) reproduced her pain with palpable crepitus.

(a) What changes are present on her lateral knee radiograph in Figure *b*?

(b) What does the skyline view show (Figure **c**)?

(c) What is the diagnosis?

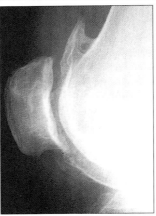

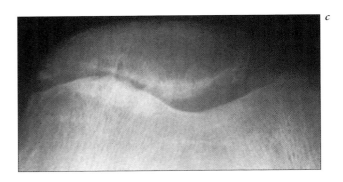

88 A 68-year-old man who had had seropositive RA for 12 years presented with a two-week history of being unable to fully extend his right ring and little fingers (Figure *a*). A simple manoeuvre gave temporary correction (Figure *b*).
(a) What is the differential diagnosis of this functional abnormality?
(b) What is the likely diagnosis?

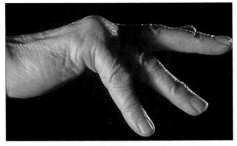

a

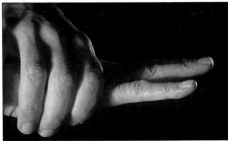

b

89 A 68-year-old patient with long-standing RA had undergone right total hip replacement seven months before referral. She now presented a three-month history of progressive right groin pain that was worse on resuming activity after rest or on rising from a chair. She was again using her walking stick, which she had discarded following her operation. Examination revealed pain on straight leg raising and tenderness over the lateral aspect of her proximal femur. All blood tests including a septic screen were negative but a technetium[99] scan showed increased activity around the prosthesis.
(a) Describe her x-ray abnormalities.
(b) What diagnoses should be considered?
(c) What further investigations, if any, are necessary?

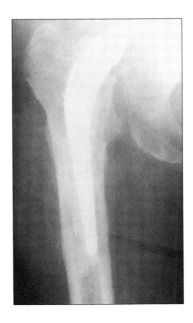

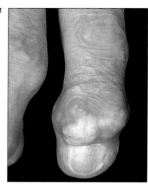
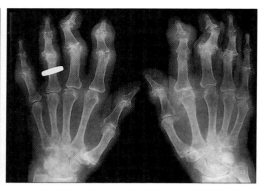

90 This 76-year-old woman had developed nodal OA in her 50s. Over the previous year she had noticed an increase in size of several of her nodes and recurrence of pain and stiffness in her interphalangeal joints. Two of her nodes had ulcerated and been treated with flucloxacillin by her GP. She was otherwise well. She had taken bendrofluazide and L-thyroxine for five years for hypertension and hypothyroidism. One of her symptomatic fingers is shown in Figure *a*.
(a) What changes are present on her hand radiograph, shown in Figure *b*?
(b) What is the diagnosis?
(c) How would you treat her?

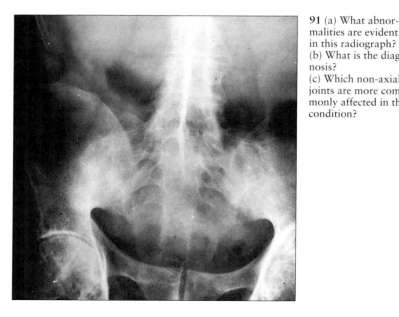

91 (a) What abnormalities are evident in this radiograph?
(b) What is the diagnosis?
(c) Which non-axial joints are more commonly affected in this condition?

92 A 65-year-old man with non-insulin dependent diabetes mellitus complained of stiff hands and increasing difficulty with precision movements. In this picture he is attempting to place his hands in the "prayer" position with wrists extended.
(a) What is the likely diagnosis?
(b) What other conditions can cause this sign?

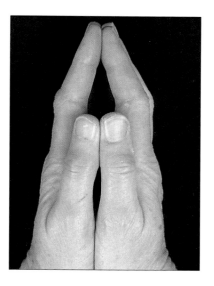

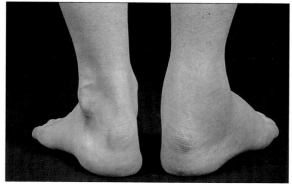

93 A 36-year-old nurse sustained a minor right ankle sprain. Over the next six weeks, however, her hindfoot and midfoot became progressively painful and swollen, as shown. Examination revealed dusky erythema, increased warmth, non-pitting oedema and diffuse tenderness. In addition, her ankle, subtalar and midtarsal movements were reduced. Routine biochemical and haematological tests, including ESR, were normal.
(a) What is the likely diagnosis?
(b) What further investigations might be helpful in confirming the diagnosis?

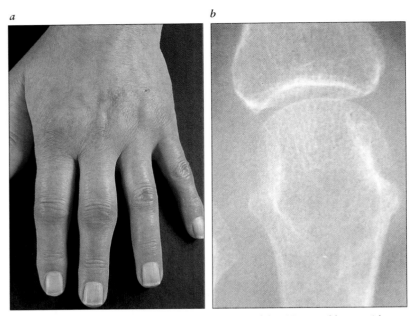

94 (a) What signs are present in the hand (Figure *a*) of this 37-year-old man with a two-year history of seropositive polyarthritis?
(b) What radiographic abnormalities are present in his middle MCPJ (Figure *b*)?

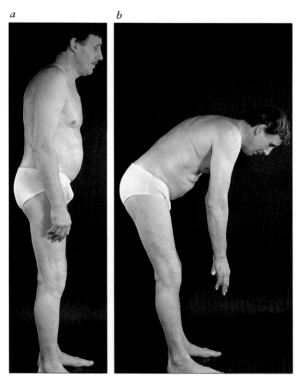

95 This patient has a long history of back pain that started
in his early twenties and requires treatment with physiotherapy, exercises and NSAIDs. He had experienced several
episodes of iritis. His father had also suffered with back
problems for many years. The patient is trying to touch his
toes (above right).
(a) What abnormalities are demonstrated in Figures *a* and *b*?
(b) What is the diagnosis?

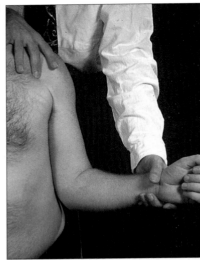

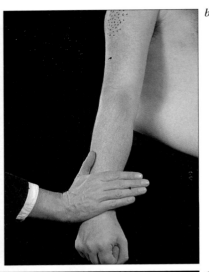

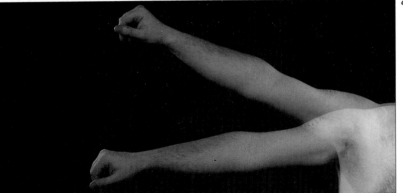

96 This 40-year-old man gave a two-month history of right upper arm pain that started after a weekend painting his ceiling. Placing his hands behind his head reproduced his pain; passive external rotation was full and pain free with no tenderness or crepitus on palpation (Figure *a*); resisted active abduction (Figure *b*) was strong but painful (site indicated by hatching); elevating his arm was painful between the two positions shown (Figure *c*).

(a) What two conditions classically cause pain limited to the arc of movement shown (above)?

(b) What is the diagnosis in this man?

97 This 73-year-old woman had an eight-year history of inflammatory arthritis principally affecting her shoulders, wrists, MCPJs, IPJs (Figure *a*) and knees (Figure *b*). She was seropositive for rheumatoid factor (Rose-Waaler and Latex but not IgG rheumatoid factor), had an elevated ESR (32mm in first hour) and had been diagnosed as RA.
(a) What features are evident on her hand radiograph (Figure *c*)?
(b) What is the diagnosis?

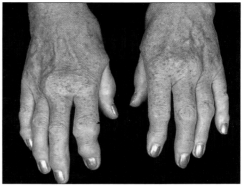

a

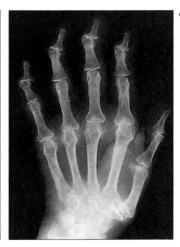

b

c

98 This 31–year–old woman has a long history of Raynaud's phenomenon, photosensitivity and arthralgia of her hands, knees and feet.
(a) What is her rash?
(b) What is her underlying diagnosis?
(c) What full blood count abnormalities commonly occur with her primary disease?

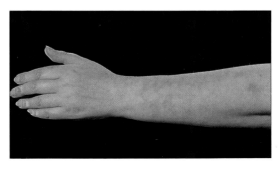

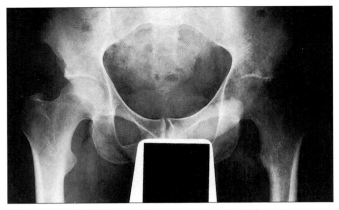

99 A previously fit 37-year-old man complained of left groin, anterior thigh and buttock pain, which had gradually developed over the previous two months. The pain was worse on weight-bearing, necessitating the use of a walking stick. There was mild early morning stiffness that persisted during rest and also disturbed his nights. He had no other joint problems and no past history of note. Examination revealed stress pain at the extremes of left hip movement and mild reduction in internal rotation.

(a) What features are shown on his x-ray?
(b) Ultrasound showed no effusion and all blood tests were normal. What is the likely diagnosis?
(c) Who is classically at risk of developing this condition?

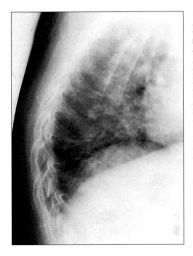

100 A 57-year-old Asian housewife presented with a six-month history of intermittent episodes of acute back pain, loss of height and increasing dorsal kyphosis. Her calcium, alkaline phosphatase, phosphate, parathormone and vitamin D levels, thyroid function, immunoglobulins, ESR and 24-hour urinary calcium excretion were normal.

(a) Describe her x-ray abnormalities.
(b) What is the likely cause of her acute painful episodes?
(c) What is her likely underlying diagnosis?

ANSWERS

1 (a) Erythema nodosum.
(b) Chest x-ray; throat swab for culture.

Erythema nodosum predominates in women, presenting as localized crops of painful red nodules with tight, shiny overlying skin. Over several days the nodules characteristically change from red to blue/yellow ("bruising" discolouration) and then resolve completely without scarring usually within three to six weeks. Crops are typically localised but occasionally widespread. Shins are the classic site but any part of the body may be involved; recurrent crops tend to affect the same site in any individual. Mild constitutional upset and arthralgia are common. As in this nurse, synovitis with marked periarticular inflammation may occur. The arthritis targets knees and ankles, less commonly involving upper limb joints; it is usually additive and eventually symmetrical.

Causes of erythema nodosum include:
common:
• acute sarcoidosis
• Streptococcal infections (the usual cause in children)
• drug reactions, eg sulphonamides, oral contraceptives
• "idiopathic" (c.15%)
uncommon:
• Crohn's disease, ulcerative colitis
• Behçet's disease
• tuberculosis
• leprosy
• acute rheumatic fever
• lymphoreticular malignancy

The chest x-ray is usually abnormal if acute sarcoidosis or tuberculosis are present. The throat is the usual site of persistent or recurrent streptococcal infection. A full history and examination usually point to drugs or less common causes and lead to targeted investigation; "blind" screening for occult triggers (eg inflammatory bowel disease) is unwarranted. An acute phase response (elevated ESR, plasma viscosity, CRP) is common during acute episodes.

Biopsy (rarely indicated) reveals non-specific inflammation with lymphocytic infiltration around septal veins in subdermal fat. Sarcoid granulomata may be present if due to sarcoid. The main differential diagnosis is from other forms of nodular panniculitis: lupus profundus (this leaves depressed scars); Weber-Christian disease; and Sweet's syndrome (prominent fever, leukocytosis, dense neutrophilic infiltration on skin biopsy). Bruising discoloration is not a feature of these rarer forms.

Treatment of an underlying cause (for this nurse antibiotics for confirmed streptococcal throat infection) is usually curative. Symptomatic treatment is with analgesics and NSAIDs. Severe or persistent episodes may warrant short-term oral steroid or a trial of dapsone.

2 (a) Olecranon bursitis.
(b) No.
(c) Trauma; sepsis; inflammatory rheumatic disease (eg RA, gout).

Bursae are fluid-filled sacs that facilitate motion between articulating structures. Their lining lacks basement membrane and resembles synovium. There are over 80 bursae each side of the body. **Subcutaneous bursae** (eg olecranon) form after birth in response to normal external friction and are non-communicating: **deep bursae** (eg subacromial) usually form before birth in response to internal movements and may communicate with joints. **Adventitious bursae** (eg over first metatarsal head) can form almost anywhere in response to abnormal shearing stress. Trauma, infection or rheumatic disease may cause inflammation (bursitis) with increased fluid production. In septic bursitis organisms are usually introduced by puncture wounds or adjacent skin cellulitis. Traumatic bursitis may be complicated by sepsis or haemorrhage. Rheumatoid or gouty nodules may occur within bursae (especially olecranon).

Olecranon bursitis causes localized swelling (transilluminable; positive balloon sign/fluctuance), warmth, tenderness and often erythema. Pain is usually minimal except when pressure is exerted (eg by tight clothing). Elbow motion is unimpaired and usually painless except in full flexion when the bursa tightens. Infection should be excluded, particularly if acute and reddened, by aspiration and examination of bursal fluid (Gram stain/culture; crystals); care must be taken not to enter the elbow capsule (risking extension of sepsis into the joint).

Non-infected bursitis usually settles if protected against additional trauma. Injection of steroid into the bursa may hasten recovery in persistant cases.

3 (a) OA.
(b) Supero-lateral, supero-medial, medial.

Radiographic features of OA at the hip, shown to varying degrees in these 3 films, include:
- joint space narrowing (usually focal)
- subchondral sclerosis (subjacent to narrowing)
- osteophyte: marginal (a)(b)(c); periosteal (inferior femoral neck "buttressing" in (a)); or central (uncommon)
- cysts (solitary acetabular cysts (b) or more widespread (c))
- femoral head migration: superior (superolateral (a); intermediate; superomedial (b)); axial; or medial
- osteochondral bodies (not shown)

Hip OA has been classified in many ways (eg "primary"versus "secondary"; "atrophic" versus "hypertrophic"), mainly on the basis of differing radiographic patterns. The pattern of femoral head migration in particular may associate with different risk factors and prognosis. For example:
superior migration:
  commonest pattern (men and women)
  mainly unilateral at presentation
  may associate with local structural abnormality (eg acetabular dysplasia, "secondary" OA)
  likely to progress (particularly superolateral)
medial migration:
  uncommon (mainly women)

more commonly bilateral at presentation
the pattern that particularly associates with nodal OA
unlikely to progress (with medial or axial migration)
   Other patterns are described (eg concentric) and many patients have "indeterminate" patterns, particularly in late, severe OA.

4 (a) Well-defined lytic lesions, with endosteal scalloping, in the femur and pubic ramus.
(b) Multiple myeloma.

In patients with regional pain, features which should alert to the possibility of malignant involvement of bone include:
• pain predominant at night ("bony pain")
• progressive pain
• pain difficult to reproduce during examination/palpation (ie explained by defined joint/periarticular problem)
• tenderness to palpation/percussion of bone (uncommon)
• weight loss
• associated symptoms/signs of primary lesion
   In this woman the distribution of pain was consistent with a hip problem. Full passive movements, however, made arthropathy very unlikely (passive and active movements are equally reduced in synovitis; at the hip stress pain occurs earliest and most severely with internal rotation in flexion). Her history of progressive night pain suggested a bone lesion; osteonecrosis usually produces usage as well as night pain, leaving tumour as the likely diagnosis. Radiographs often help in this situation, and changes in (a) were characteristic of myeloma. Pain from malignant bone deposits is often ameliorated by NSAIDs.
   Myeloma may present with locomotor symptoms due to:
• deposits in bone (as in this case)
• associated amyloid deposition
• arthritis resembling carcinoma polyarthritis
• associated sepsis (arthritis, osteomyelitis)
   Bone pain, mainly lumbar or thoracic back pain, is the commonest presentation; the hip is the commonest extra-spinal site followed by shoulder and knee. Acute pain from pathological fracture is not uncommon. Radiographs may show lytic lesions (not always hot on bone scan) or generalised osteopenia. It may occasionally cause confusion with polymyalgia rheumatica by presentation with proximal limb girdle "stiffness" and increased ESR.
   Further investigations in this woman showed elevated ESR, a monoclonal gammopathy with reduction in IgM and IgA, Bence-Jones proteinuria, and similar lytic lesions in the contralateral femur, pelvis, humeri and skull; bone marrow confirmed an IgG lamda-secreting myeloma. She received melphalan and prednisolone and her regional pain was greatly helped by radiotherapy to the left pelvis and femur.

5 (a) A large fluffy opacification in the right lower/mid zone with no cavitation. The appearance is consistent with vasculitis or infection.
(b) Wegener's granulomatosis.
(c) Oral prednisolone (daily) and cyclophosphamide (usually given weekly by oral or intravenous route, with an anti-emetic).

Wegener's granulomatosis is a rare multisystem disease that causes necrotising, granulomatous vasculitis that particularly targets the upper and lower respiratory tract, eyes and ears, and kidney. The following clinicopathological features may occur:
- paranasal sinuses (rhinorrhoea, nose-bleeds, sinus pain)
- nasopharynx (mucosal ulcers, saddle nose deformity)
- lungs (cough, chest pain, haemoptysis; granular infiltrates that may cavitate)
- eyes (kerato-conjunctivitis, sclero-uveitis, proptosis)
- ears (deafness)
- kidney (haematuria, proteinuria, renal failure; focal segmental or necrotising glomerulonephritis)
- skin (bruising, purpura, nodules, ulcers)
- joints (arthralgia, migratory polyarthritis)
- peripheral neuropathy (mononeuritis multiplex)
- heart (pericarditis, arrythmia, infarction)

Onset may be relatively acute or insidious. It predominates in middle age, and mainly affects men (2:1). The differential diagnosis may include midline granuloma, lymphomatoid granulomatosis and other forms of systemic vasculitis.

This patient had granulomatous infiltration affecting his eye and retro-orbital tissues, causing proptosis and diplopia, as well as sinus involvement (all demonstrated on CT scan). His chest radiograph showed typical patchy vasculitis, in this case with no cavitation. He had no evidence of renal involvement; this is rarely an initial manifestation but eventually develops in the majority (deterioration in renal function can be rapid, but hypertension is uncommon). His ESR was 105 with a normochromic, normocytic anaemia. He had a positive ANCA (anti neutrophil cytoplasmic antibody): examination by direct immunofluorescence showed a cytoplasmic (cANCA) rather than perinuclear (pANCA) staining pattern (high titres of cANCA particularly associate with Wegener's; the titre in an individual correlates with disease activity).

Confirmation of the diagnosis is by histology of biopsied material; the nasopharynx is the usual site (though granulomata in nasal mucosa may be hard to interpret) but in this man retrobulbar tissue was obtained.

Cyclophosphamide has been shown to be effective in reducing the high mortality associated with this condition. Prednisolone is often given initially with eye, renal or cardiac involvement. Following institution of cyclophosphamide and prednisolone this man made a full recovery with no impaired vision.

6 (a). Figure *b*: erosion, irregularity and widening of left sacroiliac joint (particularly the synovial lower two-thirds), osteopenia of sacral side.

Figure *c*: widening of left sacroiliac joint; loss of cortical integrity (particularly sacral side); sequestrum in anterior aspect of joint.
(b) Left sacroiliac joint sepsis.

Features that particularly suggest septic arthritis include:
- progressive pain (worse from week to week) with marked rest and night (not just usage) pain

- additive joint involvement in one limb (eg first MTPJ, followed by ankle, then knee)
- overlying erythema (peripheral/superficial joints)
- involvement of "odd" joints (eg single sacroiliac, sternoclavicular joint)
- disproportionate symptoms in one or a few joints in a patient with RA
- predisposing medical conditions (eg sepsis elsewhere, diabetes, leukaemia, drug abuse, AIDS)

The knee is the commonest site for sepsis, though sacroiliac and sternoclavicular joints, hip and spine are classic target sites in subjects with impaired immunity.

The distribution of this patient's referred pain (buttock, posterior thigh) was typical of sacroiliitis; its progressive nature and marked nocturnal component suggested sepsis. Although the adult sacroiliac joint is virtually immobile, standing on the ipsilateral leg or applying "stress" (Figure *a*) may reproduce the pain. Two other stress tests may be tried with the patient supine: (a) forcible downward pressure on both anterior iliac crests, or (b) flexing the ipsilateral hip and knee and pushing the knee towards the contralateral shoulder. Stress tests, however, are insensitive and imaging is the main way of demonstrating abnormality.

Although sacroiliitis in Reiter's and psoriasis may initially be unilateral, erosive changes are not as florid as in Figure *b* and usually predominate on the iliac side (cartilage is thicker on the sacral side). Furthermore, extensive osteopenia is not a feature. Demonstration of sequestrum on CT (Figure *c*) was diagnostic. The principal considerations were:
- staphylococcal infection (most likely)
- less common pyogenic bacteria (eg pseudomonas aeruginosa, streptococcus pneumoniae, fusobacterium)
- tuberculosis (usually insidious in onset)
- gonococcus (mainly targets peripheral, not axial joints)
- brucellosis (mainly targets spine >SIJs, occupational/ regional predisposition)
- fungi, opportunist infections (rare, immunocompromised patients)

Search for a primary site of infection included cultures of blood (usually positive in >50% of non-tuberculous septic arthritis), throat and nasal swabs, urine and stools; the chest x-ray was normal and a bone scan showed no other focus. Biopsy of the joint confirmed staphylococcal sepsis. Parenteral flucloxacillin (two weeks) followed by oral administration (three months) resulted in complete recovery and normalisation of his initially elevated ESR and CRP. Radiographic fusion was apparent 12 months later.

Although sepsis can occur in previously normal joints (the usual situation in children) its occurrence in adults should lead to consideration of predisposing impaired immunity. This patient denied drug abuse and had no high risk factors for AIDS; thorough clinical examination was normal. Following initial recovery his serum immunoglobulins, full blood count, ESR and complement (C3, C4) levels were normal, and he was not investigated further.

7 (a) Figure *a*: the right knee shows widening of femoral and tibial condyles; widened intercondylar notch; course trabecular pattern; obliteration of both tibiofemoral compartments; mild sclerosis. Figure *b*: posterior tibial subluxation with remodelling and a large patella.

(b) Chronic haemophilic arthropathy.

Haemarthrosis is a common presenting feature of haemophilia A (Factor VIII deficiency) and the clinically indistinguishable haemophilia B (Factor IX deficiency, Christmas disease). Both are inherited as a sex-linked recessive disorder of men. A family history is usual though not inevitable (due to a high incidence of spontaneous mutation). Presentation is usually in the first few years of life but occasionally (as in this patient) in later childhood or adolescence. The rheumatological manifestations of haemophilia are:
• acute muscle bleeds
• acute haemarthrosis
• muscle and joint contractures
• chronic haemophilic arthropathy
   Bleeding into muscle is commoner in children than adults and follows minor trauma. Flexors are most commonly affected (iliopsoas, forearm, quadriceps, calf). Bleeds may be complicated by peripheral nerve entrapment, fibrosis and contracture.
   Acute haemarthrosis is usually spontaneous and affects one joint at a time. As with any bleeding diathesis (eg anticoagulants, leukaemia) the elbows, knees and ankles are particularly targeted (interestingly all hinge joints). The patient may get a warning symptom (prickling, warmth) followed by rapid onset of pain and swelling, reaching a maximum over a few hours. Examination reveals a very tender, tensely swollen joint held in flexion; in some cases pain and muscle spasm are dominant with little joint swelling, probably due to subarticular rather than intracapsular bleeds. Treatment consists of replacement of appropriate clotting factor as soon as possible, immobilisation, ice-packs, aspiration of large tense effusions, followed by early mobilisation once the pain has subsided. Complete recovery may follow early bleeds, but with recurrent episodes chronic proliferative synovitis develops, (probably secondary to retained iron) and this, together with subarticular bleeds, produces:
• growth anomalies with enlargement of epiphyses
• articular surface damage
• chronic destructive change
   The distribution of chronic haemophilic arthropathy is the same as for acute bleeds with elbows and knees being most affected. Flexion contractures, crepitus, bony overgrowth and modest synovitis are typical findings. Particularly if there has been prior muscle or nerve damage gross crippling deformities can result ("crippling joint disease"). Acute haemarthrosis becomes less common with time but chronic destructive change is usually slowly progressive.
   The radiographic signs in this patient are typical of any inflammatory arthropathy occurring during growth (combining cartilage loss with stimulated bone growth and remodelling). Posterior tibial subluxation and fixed flexion are characteristic deformities of any juvenile chronic arthritis. Haemophilia, however, was suggested by his gender, the history of recurrent acute episodes leading onto chronic disease, and asymmetric involvement of elbows, knees and ankles.

8 (a) Loss of intervertebral height (C5/C6, C6/C7, C7/T1); minor anterior osteophyte; subluxation with anterior slippage (step-laddering) of C5 on C6; degenerative change/sclerosis of facet joints (eg C5/C6/C7).
(b) RA.
(c) RA affects the cervical spine early in its course; its severity and progression then correlate with that of peripheral joints. Atlanto-axial subluxation, not seen in this case, also usually mirrors the severity of peripheral joints.

Subaxial cervical involvement in RA is secondary to inflammatory damage to joints, bone and ligaments. The initial lesion is often synovitis of neuro-central joints which erodes adjacent disc and bone to cause subluxation, resulting in ligamentous laxity and secondary mechanical damage. Subaxial subluxations particularly target C2-C3 and C3-C4 segments, typically lack osteophytes, and are often at multiple levels, giving the "stepladder" appearance; end-plate erosions are ocasionally evident. Accompanying instability associates with a high risk of damage to nerve roots or spinal cord. Unlike seronegative spondarthropathies, the thoracic and lumbar spine are rarely affected in RA.
   Pain of cervical spine involvement is typically localized to the neck and occiput and accompanied by stiffness, reduced movement and crepitus. Cord involvement may cause pyramidal long tract signs; vertebrobasilar insufficiency may cause loss of equilibrium, tinnitus, vertigo, visual disturbances and diplopia. Subjective sensation in the limbs may be altered, with paresthesiae, numbness and "hot and cold" sensations. Bulbar disturbance can be paroxysmal and fatal, presenting as abnormalities in swallowing and phonation. Spincter disturbance must be watched for. Interpretation of symptoms and signs may be problematic in the presence of severe polyarticular disease. Loss of function may result from articular disease, neuropathy and diffuse muscle weakness in patients with RA; therefore, a high index of suspicion of cervical spine involvement is required.

9 (a) Unilateral parotid enlargement.
(b) Schirmer's test.
(c) Primary Sjögren's syndrome.

Sjögren's syndrome is an autoimmune disorder that is characterised by cellular infiltration and subsequent fibrosis and atrophy of lacrimal, salivary and other exocrine glands. It may occur alone ("primary") but more commonly associates with RA, SLE and other connective tissue diseases ("secondary"). Keratoconjunctivitis sicca or ocular dryness may be asymptomatic or cause burning and itchiness (occasionally paradoxical watering of eyes), often with sticky, inspissated, rope-like material in the inner canthus. Sicca syndrome is screened for by the Schirmer Tear Test in which a strip of filter paper is looped over the outer third of the lower eyelid. A normal test results in wetting of the paper greater than 10mm in five minutes. Between 5 and 10mm is considered equivocal and <5mm abnormal. The test is commonly positive in otherwise normal elderly subjects. Confirmation of the syndrome is by Rose Bengal staining and slit-lamp examination, which shows uptake of stain in damaged corneal epithelium, filamentary keratitis and occasionally corneal ulceration. Other tear tests (eg tear-film break-up, lysozyme activity) are also commonly abnormal.

Salivary gland inflammation and atrophy results in a dry mouth (xerostomia) and difficulty in forming a bolus. Tongue fissuring, dental caries and angular cheilosis may also occur. The patient often takes frequent drinks of water throughout the night. Parotid enlargement may be noted during the inflammatory phase but is rarely persistent. Sialography may show dilated parotid ducts, and duct atrophy and other tests of salivary activity may also be positive. Although invasive, a labial (lip) gland biopsy is simple to perform and will provide definite evidence of focal lymphocyte infiltration, acinar atrophy, fibrofatty replacement (+/-proliferation of myoepithelial cells or ducts) in patients with Sjögren's.

Other occasional features of Sjögren's syndrome include:
• atrophic vaginitis (pruritus, dyspareunia, secondary infections)
• lethargy, fatiguability
• Raynaud's disease, arthralgia, myositis
• splenomegaly, widespread lymphadenopathy
• peripheral sensory neuropathy
• renal tubular acidosis, pancreatitis, basal atelectasis, thyroiditis, meningism (though these are rare)

Laboratory findings may include mild anaemia and leucopenia, elevated ESR, a polyclonal rise in immunoglobulins (especially IgA), and positive rheumatoid and antinuclear factors. Ro (SSA) and La (SSB) antibodies are both present in most cases (antisalivary antibodies in 50% of cases).

Other causes of salivary gland enlargement should be considered eg tumour (including lymphoma), sarcoidosis and mumps. Non-Hodgkins lymphoma may rarely complicate Sjögren's; this is heralded by persistent parotid swelling, lymphadenopathy, splenomegaly and fall in previously elevated serum IgM and RhF levels.

Steroids or cytotoxics may benefit systemic upset and gland swelling. Dry-eye symptoms and complications (infection, corneal scarification) are helped by regular application of "artificial tear" eye drops (eg hypomellose); cauterisation of the lacrimal puncta and canaliculi is reserved for resistant cases. Artificial saliva spray often helps xerostomia.

10 (a) Unilateral (left) sacroiliitis; irregular erosion and sclerosis both sides of the sacroiliac joint (SIJ), and widening of joint space.
(b) Chronic Reiter's disease.

Radiographic changes at the SIJ may be difficult to interpret, especially in adolescents and young adults when joint irregularity and ill-defined margins may be normal. The joint follows an oblique course and no single x-ray view looks through its entire length; an antero-posterior view shows both anterior and posterior margins and is sufficient for most purposes. The lower two-thirds of the SIJ is diarthrodial (synovial), whereas the upper third is fibrous.

This patient has unilateral sacroiliitis predominantly affecting the lower, synovial portion of the joint. His buttock pain with radiation posteriorly down the thigh ("sciatica") fits well with sacroiliac pain; in contrast to root entrapment SIJ pain does not radiate beyond the knee. Stress tests of the SIJ are insensitive and often negative (as in this case). Infection may produce unilateral sacroiliitis but would normally associate with progressive pain and radiographic osteopenia, more florid erosion and less sclerosis. Sacroiliitis due to seronegative spondarthropathy is more likely. Psoriasis and Reiter's typically produce unilateral, asymmetric sacroiliitis (cf bilateral, symmetrical sacroiliitis in classic ankylosing spondylitis and inflammatory bowel disease). The concurrence of plantar fasciitis and previous history of self-limiting asymmetrical lower limb synovitis, and absence of skin disease or nail dystrophy favour chronic Reiter's disease. The triad of arthritis, urethritis and conjunctivitis in acute Reiter's syndrome is often incomplete and the previous history of arthritis only in this man is not inconsistent with the diagnosis. No clear history of the triggering infection to reactive arthritis (urethritis, dysentery) is also common. Occult Crohn's disease might be considered, though unilateral sacroiliitis and peripheral enthesopathy would be atypical.

11 (a) Gross generalised osteopenia of left hand; marked cartilage and bone attrition in the carpus with loss of cortical outline.
(b) Cholesterol crystals.
(c) Chronic infection; tuberculosis.

Cholesterol crystals are a non-specific synovial fluid finding. They particularly occur in chronically inflamed joints with poor lymphatic drainage and clearance of cellular debris.

When a patient presents with inflammatory monoarthritis it is important to remember that some polyarticular conditions may have a predominantly monoarticular onset; lesser degrees of joint involvement may have gone unnoticed and a full clinical examination is required. Common conditions in which this may arise include:
• RA (a small proportion but numerically important)
• psoriatic arthritis
• Reiter's syndrome
• ankylosing spondylitis
• pyrophosphate arthropathy
• juvenile chronic arthritis
    Once established that the patient has a true chronic inflammatory monoarthritis the following may require consideration:
• chronic infection – particularly tuberculosis and atypical mycobacteria (rarely fungi, brucella, syphilis)
• sarcoidosis
• foreign bodies (eg plant-thorns, prosthetic particles)
• proliferative disorders (pigmented villonodular synovitis, osteochondromatosis, tumours)
• relapsing polychondritis (very rare)
• Familial Mediterranean fever (very rare)
    Some of these conditions favour certain joint sites (eg knee and ankle in sarcoid). Radiography is a useful first investigation and often gives specific clues, as in this patient.
    Tuberculous arthritis is most commonly mono- or oligo-articular with particular predilection in adults for the spine (especially thoracic). In children hip involvement is more usual. It may occur at any age but is most

common in children, the elderly, and the Asian community. Onset is often insidious and symptoms may predate diagnosis by several years. Examination often shows relatively modest inflammatory signs for the degree of structural damage. Radiographs of peripheral joints show focal and later regional osteopenia, cartilage loss (early), and "moth-eaten" indistinct bone outlines (with occasional clear erosions) and destructive change. In the spine spondylodiscitis (disc space narrowing with erosion and irregularity of adjacent vertebral end-plates) progresses classically in an anterior-posterior direction, with vertical spread to adjacent vertebrae along the anterior longitudinal ligament (often with gross soft tissue swelling; Question and Answer No. **89**); classic anterior wedging may subsequently develop (Pott's disease with gibbus).

Other TB foci (mainly chest, lymph node) are detected in 50%.

Confirmation is by histology and culture of synovial fluid and tissue; characteristic caseating granulomata may be obtained but positive culture is specific. Antituberculous drugs readily access bone and joints and combination chemotherapy is given (minimum 6 months) as for pulmonary TB. Surgical intervention may be required for neurological complications from spinal instability. Healing is often followed by bony ankylosis.

This patient made an excellent symptomatic and functional recovery on rifampicin, isoniazid and pyrazinamide for two months, followed by rifampacin and isoniazid for 4 months.

12 (a) Figure *a*: fibrosing alveolitis (interstitial fibrosis) with diffuse reticular lower zone shadowing. Figure *b*: cavitating nodule (left lower zone).
(b) Pleural disease (effusion, empyema); pneumonitis; vasculitis; airways disease; drug complications.

Interstitial fibrosis results from increase in mesenchymal cells. Classical signs are showers of end-inspiratory crackles predominating in lower zones. Radiographs may show diffuse reticular or reticulo-nodular shadowing, later merging into a classic honeycomb appearance. Pulmonary function tests show a restrictive pattern with decreased diffusion capacity; biopsy shows diffuse fibrosis and variable mononuclear infiltrate. Smoking associates with a higher prevalence of fibrosis (and bronchiectasis). Patients are often asymptomatic and the outcome generally good. Rarely, presentation is with breathlessness, clubbing, cyanosis and active desquamative interstitial pneumonitis: such symptomatic patients usually have progressive respiratory failure and high mortality.

Intrapulmonary rheumatoid nodules may be single or multiple, usually appearing round or lobulated. They may occur anywhere but predominate in upper zones. They do not invade adjacent tissue or cause distal collapse. They may come and go spontaneously or cavitate and result in bronchopleural fistula; they may rarely predate the arthritis. Especially with single lesions alternative coexistent causes (carcinoma, abscess, hamartoma) need exclusion; this often requires biopsy (coexistent nodules and carcinoma are reported). Caplans syndrome is coexistent RA and pneumoconiosis (coalminers) in which aggressive fibroblastic reaction results in dramatic obliterative granulomatous fibrosis.

Pleural disease in RA is discussed elsewhere. Arteritis may rarely involve the pulmonary vasculature, causing pulmonary infarction and even pulmonary hypertension.

Reduced maximum expiratory flow rate and forced expiratory volume occur more commonly in RA patients (c.50%) than controls (c.20%). A number of drugs used to treat RA may result in parenchymal disease (eg methotrexate, azathioprine, gold, chlorambucil); NSAIDs may exacerbate or provoke asthma.

13 (a) Figure *a*: Barium meal showing dilatation of jejenum and duodenum with "wire spring"(stack of coins) appearance, flocculation of barium and numerous diverticuli. Figure *b*: Barium swallow showing decreased peristalsis, dilatation and ulceration of the distal oesophagus.

(b) Systemic sclerosis (scleroderma).

After skin changes and Raynaud's phenomenon gut involvement is the commonest manifestation of scleroderma. Identical oesophageal involvement – a principal feature of CREST (calcinosis, Raynaud's, esophageal, telangiectasia) syndrome – occurs with limited and diffuse/systemic scleroderma. Impaired lower esophageal mobility and sphincter dysfunction cause acid reflux with heartburn, dysphagia or odynophagia (pain on swallowing). Dysfunction results from a combination of ischaemic nerve damage, inflammation and fibrosis. Complications of chronic reflux include erosive oesophagitis, Barretts esophagus, stricture and aspiration. NSAIDs may contribute. Oesophageal dysfunction and oesophagitis are common even in asymptomatic patients.

Stomach involvement is unusual, though gastric outlet obstruction and bleeding (from telangiectasia, NSAIDs) may occur. Small bowel dysfunction is very common (c.50%) resulting in fibrosis, smooth muscle dysfunction/atrophy and diverticuli. Symptoms include abdominal bloating, cramps and diarrhoea. Malabsorption, due to fibrosis or secondary bacterial overgrowth, is uncommon; pneumatosis intestinalis cystoides, volvulus and perforation are rare.

Colonic involvement occurs in most patients. Though usually asymptomatic, constipation, obstruction and pseudo-obstruction may result from abnormal motility. Wide-mouthed diverticuli along the anti-mesenteric border are characteristic but rarely cause complications (bleeding, perforation, abscess).

For oesophageal involvement the following advice/interventions may be relevant:

• avoid large meals
• avoid post-prandial recumbancy
• wear loose clothing
• stop smoking
• regular antacids
• H_2 blockers, gaviscon, omeprazole
• metoclopramide (aids oesophageal mobility)

- dilatation, surgery (for stricture)

Small bowel involvement may require broad spectrum antibiotics. Constipation is managed with bulking and softening agents.

14 (a) Bright red discoloration due to prominent corneal vessels (individual vessels clearly seen), sparing the limbus and diffusely affecting both eyes. (b) Episcleritis.

Episcleritis is common in RA, particularly women. It affects the anterior sclera, usually close to the limbus. Episcleritis may be localized or diffuse, often bilateral, typically appearing as raised lesions a few millimetres in diameter surrounded by intense hyperemia of superficial vessels. It may cause minor discomfort but pain is not prominent. The eyes are flushed bright red and individual vessels are clearly seen. In contrast to conjunctivitis the vessels cannot be moved over the surface of the eyeball but will constrict with adrenaline eye-drops. Episcleritis is usually transient but may persist for weeks or months. It does not associate with severe systemic disease.

Scleritis is much less common. It is often accompanied by episcleritis but is a serious condition requiring urgent treatment (oral steroids). Scleritis is usually painful (sometimes severe) and the deep scleral vessels impart a dark purple hue in contrast to the red flush of episcleritis; deep vessels do not constrict with adrenaline drops. Nodular scleritis results in a localized, painful, congested area raised due to scleral oedema; inflammation alters scleral proteoglycans so that the sclera becomes transparent, permitting the dark choroid to be seen. Diffuse scleritis is less severe but inflammation may involve the cornea, causing keratitis and keratolysis ("corneal melt"). Necrotising scleritis is rare; granulomatous nodules may result in perforation (scleromalacia perforans). Posterior scleritis is difficult to diagnose because there is nothing visibly amiss; instead there may be pain and visual disturbance from retinal detachment caused by the intense inflammatory exudation.

Corneal and conjunctival manifestations of sicca syndrome are the commonest opthalmological features of RA. Drug-related ocular disorders are rare but include gold deposition in the cornea, corneal and retinal changes related to antimalarials, and posterior subcapsular cataracts caused by corticosteroids. Another rare complication is Brown's Syndrome, with diplopia on upward and inward gaze, caused by tenovaginitis of the superior oblique tendon.

15 (a) Increased interosseous distance ("joint space") in both tibiofemoral compartments; "squaring" of femoral and tibial condyles; prominent fibular head.
(b) Acromegalic arthropathy.

Rheumatic complaints occur in the majority of acromegalics and may be the presenting feature. Common problems include:
- low back pain (due to hypermobility)
- carpal tunnel syndrome (usually bilateral)
- acromegalic arthropathy (mainly symptomic at knees)
- Raynaud's phenomenon

Rheumatic syndromes to particularly consider in renal dialysis patients include:
- azotaemic osteoarthropathy
- acute calcific periarthritis (apatite crystal deposition)
- acute and chronic gout (urate crystal deposition)
- pyrophosphate arthropathy (calcium pyrophosphate crystal deposition)
- "osteogenic" synovitis due to hyperparathyroidism
- avascular necrosis
- septic arthritis (often with atypical organisms)

21 (a) Ankle synovitis/effusion; valgus subtalar deformity; loss of transverse and longitudinal arches; some spreading of the toes ("daylight sign") resulting from MTPJ disease.
(b) Tibialis posterior; arising from the interosseous membrane and posterior surfaces of the tibia and fibula it angles behind and below the medial malleolus (beneath the flexor retinaculum) and inserts into the navicular, inner cuneiform and by slips to the middle three phalanges. It plantar flexes and inverts the foot.

RA may affect the ankle (talocrural), subtalar or midtarsal joints in addition to target MTPJs. Tendon sheaths of tibialis posterior (medial), peroneus brevis and longus (lateral) and tibialis anterior, extensor hallucis longus and extensor digitorum longus (anterior) are commonly involved, occasionally with rupture. Prominent medial and lateral swellings at the ankle are commonly due to tendon sheath inflammation (ankle synovitis causes anterior and posterior swelling). The Achilles tendon may be involved and is a common site for nodules. Severe ankle involvement is relatively uncommon. The subtalar joint, however, is the target joint in the hindfoot and chronic disease typically results in valgus deformity and loss of arches. In severe cases this may cause the fibula to abut onto the calcaneus resulting in stress fracture of the lower fibula. Midtarsal disease may result in a relatively rigid flat foot, making walking on uneven surfaces particularly difficult. MTPJ involvement commonly causes the sensation of "walking on pebbles".
Once established, hindfoot deformity, as in this case, is managed orthotically (eg medial arch support; thick, shock-absorbing soles).

22 (a) A large irregular soft tissue swelling extending along the little toe; pressure erosion of the proximal phalanx shaft (and to a lesser extent the metacarpal); retained joint space/contour.
(b) Pigmented villonodular synovitis (PVNS) of extensor digitorum longus tendon sheath.
(c) Knee.

PVNS is a chronic inflammatory tumorous lesion of unknown aetiology, resembling most closely a benign neoplasm. It may involve the lining of joints, bursae or tendon sheaths, causing local destruction but rarely metastasising. Lesions may be diffuse or localised and consist of villous and nodular growths within a thin layer of synovial lining cells. The central stroma contains heterogeneous cells (lipid-laden foam cells, haemosiderin-containing cells, multinucleate giant cells), collagen bundles and blood vessels. Early lesions are highly vascular. Depending on cell predominance lesions vary in colour from yellow (lipid) to dark brown (haemosiderin). Bone involvement can result from direct penetration or from mass pressure effects (as in this case).

PVNS is usually unifocal, with tenosynovium particularly targeted. After ganglia, PVNS is the commonest soft tissue tumour of the hand. The knee is the commonest joint, though any limb joint may be affected. There is no systemic upset or acute phase response. Presentation is with mild pain and gradual increase in swelling. X-rays show increased synovial mass (synovium and fluid); characteristically osteopenia and calcification are absent. Cystic bony lesions (multiple, one or both sides of the joint) may occur; the tighter the capsule the earlier cysts develop. Arthrography demonstrates recesses and filling defects. MRI is now the investigation of choice but histology is required for diagnosis.

Treatment is usually by open or arthroscopic excision (other approaches include intra-articular radiocolloid, external beam radiotherapy). Recurrence usually only occurs with PVNS affecting the knee. Chronic pain and limited joint motion are frequent chronic sequelae.

23 (a) Chondrocalcinosis of wrist triangular ligament and knee fibro- and hyaline cartilage.
(b) Serum magnesium, calcium, alkaline phosphatase, and ferritin. Synovial fluid examination for calcium pyrophosphate (CPPD) crystals.

Chondrocalcinosis (cartilage calcification) usually results from deposition of CPPD crystals (rarely apatite and other basic calcium phosphates). CPPD deposition is a common, predominantly age-related phenomenon that may occur in normal cartilage (isolated chondrocalcinosis) or in association with osteoarthritis (chronic "pyrophosphate arthropathy"). In both instances "shedding" of CPPD crystals from preformed cartilage deposits can produce attacks of florid synovitis ("pseudogout"). Attacks are self-limiting over one to three weeks and commonly associate with erythema and desquamation.

CPPD crystals preferentially deposit in fibrocartilage (knee menisci, triangular ligament, symphysis pubis) and hyaline cartilage (especially knee), but may also cause calcification of capsule, ligaments, and tendons (bursal and soft tissue deposits are rare). The knee, wrist and symphysis are the commonest sites for radiographic chondrocalcinosis, followed by shoulders, hips, elbows and spine (other sites are rare).

Associations of CPPD and chondrocalcinosis include:
• ageing
• familial predisposition
• metabolic disease
• joint insult, OA
(a negative association occurs with RA)
Chondrocalcinosis is rare under age 55, but increases in prevalence from c.5% in the seventh decade to c.30% in those over 80. Premature-onset chondrocalcinosis, particularly polyarticular, should lead to consideration of metabolic or familial predisposition. Predisposing metabolic diseases include:
• hyperparathyroidism

- haemochromatosis
- hypomagnesaemia
- hypophosphatasia

Aspiration of knee fluid in this patient confirmed CPPD crystals. Screening revealed hypomagnesaemia subsequently shown to result from an isolated renal tubular defect (with mild hypokalaemia but not Barter's syndrome). First degree relatives were found to be unaffected. She was given oral magnesium carbonate supplementation with partial correction serum levels and reduction in frequency of acute attacks. Her radiographic chondrocalcinosis appeared unchanged after five years.

24 (a) "Sausage digit".
(b) Soft-tissue swelling of IPJ, joint-space loss, erosion with fluffy new bone formation expanding the phalanx base ("proliferative erosion"), and retained bone density.
(c) Psoriatic arthropathy.

Combined swelling of interphalangeal joints and soft tissues, including flexor tendon sheaths, of a digit ("sausage digit") is highly characteristic of psoriatic arthropathy, even in the absence of skin or nail lesions (it also occurs in Reiter's syndrome). Such swelling contrasts with finger "spindling" in RA. Fingers and toes are equally affected but usually only one or a few digits are involved synchronously. Onset is often abrupt. Symptoms and swelling usually last several months but commonly subside with mild or no disability.

Radiographic features are often equally characteristic and include:
- relative absence of periarticular osteoporosis
- erosions combined with new bone response ("proliferative erosion") affecting joints (giving a "mouse-ear" appearance at IPJs) and entheses, eg around the calcaneus
- proliferative periostitis/osteitis, producing a white "ivory phalanx"
- tendency to fibrosis/ankylosis
- whittling of terminal phalangeal tufts – acro-osteolysis (uncommon)

Asymptomatic sacroiliitis (commonly asymmetric, unilateral) may additionally be present. Severe deforming arthritis with bone resorption (arthritis mutilans) and extensive spondylitis may occur in patients with psoriasis. However, those with sausage digits usually have a good prognosis, the principal other joint involvement being intermittent oligoarticular synovitis (particularly of the knees).

25 (a) Dermatomyositis associated with colonic neoplasm.
(b) Muscle enzymes (eg creatine kinase); muscle biopsy; electromyography.

The association of adult polymyositis (c.10%) with malignancy (particularly lung, gastrointestinal tract, breast, uterus, ovary, nasopharynx) is poorly understood. Myositis may precede, coincide or follow other features of the malignancy. The association predominates in the middle-aged and is highest in men over age 50 with dermatomyositis (c.60%). In practice limited screening for occult malignancy is warranted in patients over 50. The dominant feature of polymyositis is muscle weakness; usually symmetrical, targeting proximal lower and upper limb muscles, trunk and neck. Problems with stairs, rising from chairs or combing hair are characteristic; marked pelvic girdle involvement may cause a waddling (bilateral Trendelenburg) gait. Dysphagia, regurgitation or dysphonia may occur with bulbar muscle involvement; significant respiratory embarrassment is uncommon and ocular muscles are spared. Muscle tenderness and pain are common accompaniments; advanced cases may show wasting. Arthralgia and synovitis may occur, though more commonly in association with underlying (eg "mixed") connective tissue disease.

The characteristic rash of dermatomyositis comprises an erythematous base with purplish, slightly raised plaques (Gottron's papules) over extensor surfaces of finger joints (Figure *a*), elbows, knees or ankles; it often resembles psoriasis. Nailfold hyperaemia with dilated capillary loops is a common accompaniment. The classical heliotrope rash with periorbital oedema is uncommon. The rash may predate muscle weakness by months, occasionally years. Pulmonary fibrosis (associating with anti Jo-1 antibodies) and cardiac abnormalities (eg heart block) are uncommon.

Muscle enzymes (creatine kinase, aldolase, lactate dehydrogenase, aspartate aminotransferase) are usually greatly elevated. Electromyography may show abnormal potentials (short duration, low amplitude, polyphasic) and fibrillation potentials at rest. Needle muscle biopsy reveals mixed fibre necrosis/regeneration and perivascular/interstitial infiltrates. Raised ESR/viscosity are usual. Non-specific auto-antibodies are common; anti Jo-1 is the most specific for polymyositis and overlap syndromes. Serial biopsies or creatine kinase levels are particularly useful as indices of treatment success.

Myositis and rash may improve following successful tumour removal/treatment. Cytotoxics (eg methotrexate, cyclophosphamide), initially combined with high-dose steroids, are the principal treatment. Not surprisingly the prognosis is worse in those patients with malignancy (due to the malignancy rather than muscle disease).

26 (a) Anterior and posterior fusion, osteopenia and underdevelopment of upper cervical vertebrae (Figure *a*); cartilage loss, coarse trabeculation, widened intercondylar notch, large patella, and abnormal bone contours at the knee (Figure *b*).
(b) Previous juvenile chronic arthritis (JCA) of polyarticular onset; now with probable secondary mechanical symptoms.

Accelerated epiphyseal maturation (increased growth but premature fusion) is common in JCA. This may result in elongation (especially of the femur) or shortening (especially of the fingers/toes); leg length discrepancy; broadened, coarse bone ends with abnormal, flattened contours; and large patellae. Radiographic erosion is uncommon and cartilage loss is usually a late radiographic feature (early non-specific features include soft-tissue swelling, osteopenia, periostitis, and delayed appearance of ossification centres). The upper/mid cervical spine (C2-5) is a target site and apophyseal joint involvement commonly leads to fusion and underdevelopment of upper segments (Figure *b*). Temporomandibular joint involvement may cause poorly differentiated condyles, limited excursion, shortened mandible (micrognathia), and malocclusion; with cervical spine fusion this may result in a characteristic bird-like facies. Subluxation of joints, particularly hips (protrusio) and knees (posterior tibial subluxation) may eventually develop. Inflammatory features may diminish in teenage- or adulthood and be followed by predominant mechanical problems (as in this case).

Diagnostic criteria for JCA (juvenile rheumatoid arthritis, or JRA in the USA) are:
- onset under 16 years
- persistent arthritis in one or more joints:
  four or less – oligoarticular
  five or more – polyarticular
- duration of three months or longer (JCA, Europe).
  six weeks or longer (JRA, USA)
- exclusion of other specific causes of arthritis in childhood.

27 (a) Viscous, clear, hyaluronate-rich "jelly".
(b) Early nodal generalised OA (NGOA).

NGOA is characterized by:
- polyarticular interphalangeal involvement of fingers
- Heberden's and Bouchard's nodes
- female preponderance
- peak onset in middle age
- good functional outcome
- predisposition to OA of knee, hip, spine
- familial predisposition

Onset is typically in the forties or fifties ("menopausal arthritis") with discomfort followed by swelling of one or a few finger interphalangeal joints. A few months later another joint becomes painful, then another – a stuttering-onset polyarthritis of interphalangeal joints ("monoarthritis multiplex"). Affected joints may show reduced movement, stress pain (limited to extremes of movement), and posterolateral swelling with occasional overlying erythema. These swellings may occur a little distance away from the joint and result from mucoid transformation of periarticular fibroadipose (some communicate with the joint). Symptoms at each joint are typically episodic for a few years, but then subside leaving firm posterolateral Heberden's (distal) and Bouchard's (proximal) nodes, lateral subluxations of interphalangeal joints, and radiographic evidence of osteoarthritis. The prognosis is excellent; hand symptoms and function two to three decades later are usually no worse than in patients with no hand OA.

28 Roth spots (cytoid bodies) and Libman-Sacks (verrucous) endocarditis.

Cytoid bodies (c.10% of patients) occur during active disease and disappear during remission. They are retinal exudates appearing as hard, white lesions adjacent to vessels. They may associate with organic brain disease and seizures. They are not disease specific and also occur in hypertensive retinopathy. Other ocular manifestations in SLE include:
- conjunctivitis or episcleritis (c.20%)
- periorbital oedema
- subconjunctival haemorrhage
- central retinal artery occlusion

SLE may cause disease of the pericardium, myocardium, endocardium and coronary arteries. Pericarditis is most common (c.30% of SLE patients) and may be asymptomatic or cause mild symptoms with an intermittent friction rub and ECG abnormalities; large pericardial effusions are rare. Myocarditis is less common and may occur in the context of vasculitis. Aortic and mitral insufficiency may result from scarring of leaflets or thickening and rupture of chordae. Verrucous endocarditis is a very common finding in patients dying of SLE. Most of these lesions (characterised by haematoxylin bodies) are microscopic; macroscopic lesions (figure *b*) are less common. Usually a pathological diagnosis, they do not associate with heart murmurs but may predispose to thrombus formation. Other cardiovascular problems include:
- Raynaud's phenomenon (20%)
- thrombosis: associated with antiphospholipid antibodies (lupus anticoagulant, anti-cardiolipin antibodies).
- cryoglobulinemia
- pulmonary hypertension
- thrombotic thrombocytopenic purpura (rare)

29 (a) Fibromyalgia syndrome.
(b) Full blood count; ESR; thyroid function; antinuclear factor; calcium.

Fibromyalgia syndrome (FS) is a common condition that predominates in middle-aged women. Principal symptoms include:
- locomotor pain – usually axial, but often felt "all over", unresponsive to analgesics, NSAIDs
- subjective morning stiffness/swelling (hands, knees)
- fatiguability – often disabling
- bifrontal and occipital headaches
- intermittent abdominal pain and altered bowel habit
- urinary frequency, dyspareunia, dysmenorrhoea
- disturbed sleep pattern, awakening unrefreshed
- irritability, weepiness, poor concentration

Symptoms are often aggravated by cold and emotional upset. Marked disability is usual; though able to wash and dress unassisted patients are often unable to do their job or routine chores. Examination is normal apart from presence of hyperalgesia at multiple tender sites, including:
- lower cervical and lumbar interspinous ligaments
- mid-supraspinatus
- mid-trapezius
- 1–2cm distal to lateral epicondyle
- second costochondral junctions
- gluteal (upper outer quadrant of buttock)
- greater trochanter
- medial fat pad at knee
- skinfold rolling over mid trapezius

Criteria for FS require hyperalgesia at tender sites (>10) axially and in both arms and legs, with negative control sites (eg distal forearm, forehead). If the patient is tender all over fabrication or psychological disturbance should be considered. FS may occur on its own (primary) but the presence of a second clinical disorder does not exclude the diagnosis.

Depending on the predominant presenting feature the patient may be labelled as having fibromyalgia, chronic fatigue syndrome, irritable bowel syndrome, tension headaches, urethral syndrome, or anxiety and depression with somatisation. There is marked overlap between these conditions, implying a spectrum of "functional" disturbance with no apparent structural, metabolic or inflammatory abnormality. FS strongly associates with sleep disturbance, specifically reduction in deep, non rapid eye movement sleep. Although the mechanisms are unclear, a simple construct is that pain or anxiety may interrupt deep, normally refreshing sleep to result in widespread interference with normal body functioning (equivalent to being "jet-lagged").

A detailed history and examination are required to exclude overt inflammatory, metabolic or endocrine disease. The principal differential diagnosis is hypothyroidism, hyperparathyroidism and lupus, justifying the investigations listed. Management involves (a) an adequate explanation to the patient, (b) strategies to increase aerobic fitness, (c) limited trial of low-dose amitriptyline (25–75mg nocte), and (d) coping strategies (eg meditational yoga). The prognosis is often poor, particularly if a specific triggering factor (commonly suppressed anxiety relating to a life event such as bereavement, marital disharmony) cannot be identified and remedied by effective counselling.

30 (a) Apatite-associated destructive arthritis; avascular necrosis; atrophic Charcot joint; sepsis.
(b) Calcific (apatite) particles and debris.
(c) Apatite-associated destructive arthritis.

Apatite (basic calcium phosphate) associated destructive arthritis (AADA; "Milwaukee shoulder syndrome") is an uncommon condition virtually restricted to elderly women. It targets hips, shoulders and knees and clinically is characterised by:
• rapid progression of pain (usage, rest and night pain)
• large, relatively cool effusions
• rapid development of marked instability
• poor outcome (usually requiring early joint replacement)

Aspirated fluid is usually non-inflammatory but contains numerous calcific particles, visible on staining with alizarin red S (a non-specific calcium stain). These particles also occur in abundance in synovium (Figure *c*). Their role in the arthropathy is unclear; their presence is non-specific, the vast quantity in AADA possibly reflecting the rapidity of bone attrition.

The radiographic features (Figures *a* and *b*) include:
• marked cartilage and bone attrition (both sides of joint)
• paucity of osteophyte and cysts ("atrophic")
• apparent increase in joint space (particularly hip, knee)
• occasional fine calcific debris

Differentiation is principally from avascular necrosis (this initially affects one side of the joint, though late necrosis may appear identical) and atrophic Charcot arthropthy (neurology in AADA is normal). Sepsis may also require consideration, but often associates with osteopenia, cortical erosion, and raised ESR. Although classified by some as a crystal deposition disease, it is often regarded as a rapidly progressive subset within the umbrella of OA.

31 (a) Rheumatoid nodules in the Achilles tendon; "cock-up" toe deformities.

(b) Rheumatoid nodules on the forearm and in association with olecranon bursitis. The nodules are firm and attached to deep structures or the wall of bursae. Bursitis is fluctuant, may transilluminate, and is not fixed to deep structures.

(c) A necrotic core of collagen fragments, fibrin, or cell debris (fibrinoid necrosis), surrounded by a radially arranged pallisade of mononuclear cells and occasional giant cells, and an outer layer of plasma cells, lymphocytes, and fibroblasts.

Rheumatoid nodules are found adjacent to and distant from articular structures. They may be subcutaneous, intracutaneous, subperiosteal, or deep inside organs (eg lungs, all layers of the heart, sclera, and meninges). Cutaneous nodules eventually occur in c.20% of patients with classic RA, targeting readily traumatised extensor surfaces with little soft tissue protection (eg elbows, forearms, wrist, MCPJs, knees, Achilles tendon, occiput, and buttocks). Other causes of nodules (gouty tophi, xanthomata, rheumatic fever, and SLE) target these same sites and histological confirmation is occasionally required for diagnosis.

Rheumatoid nodules form around areas of local vasculitis and trauma; "cropping" of plentiful nodules may accompany systemic vasculitis, the nodules sometimes ulcerating and becoming secondarily infected. Rheumatoid patients with nodules are invariably seropositive for rheumatoid factor. Nodules rarely cause pressure erosions of underlying bone; they do not calcify but may undergo necrobiosis and appear as cystic swellings. Occasionally nodules in the sclera (nodular scleritis) may lead to perforation. Troublesome nodules (eg those causing pain because of their position) may regress rapidly when injected with a steroid.

32 (a) Left-sided sacroiliitis (widening, erosion and sclerosis both sides of the joint); dilated loops of bowel, particularly transverse colon, with loss of haustral pattern.

(b) Inflammatory bowel disease (probably ulcerative colitis (UC)); early ankylosing spondylitis (AS).

AS and inflammatory bowel disease (UC, Crohn's) are disease associations, AS in association with UC/Crohn's being indistinguishable from sporadic AS. AS occurs in 15% of patients with UC. The 2 diseases run independent clinical courses and may be separated in onset by years. By contrast "enteropathic arthropathy", which particularly targets knees and ankles, mirrors the inflammatory activity of the bowel disease. It is more common in Crohn's (20%) than UC (10%) but is the commonest extra-colonic manifestation of childhood UC. Synovitis is acute, often peaking within several days and involving only one or a few joints; occasionally more joints may become involved in migratory fashion. Erythema nodosum may accompany the arthropathy. In most cases attacks are quickly self-limiting as bowel symptoms are brought under control; arthritis may rarely persist for months or years but erosion or structural damage is not a feature. Most episodes occur during the first years of the disease; remission after colectomy is usual.

Sacroiliitis in AS often gives few or no symptoms; radiographic changes are typically bilateral and symmetrical in established AS but may be asymmetric in early disease (as in this man). Infective dysentery is a possibility in this patient (as a primary problem or exacerbating trigger to UC); however, in reactive arthritis triggered by dysentery peripheral arthritis predominates (absent in this man) and florid radiographic sacroiliitis is not a feature in the acute stage. Sacroiliac joint sepsis would be expected to give progressive, severe buttock pain and a different x-ray appearance (osteopenia, predominant erosive change, less sclerosis).

NSAIDs may exacerbate UC and should be used with caution. Sulphasalazine and cytotoxics (eg azathioprine) are used to control inflammation in both UC and AS.

33 Plant-thorn synovitis.

Sharp hard plant-thorns readily penetrate skin, synovium, tendon sheath, or periosteum. Plant-thorn fragments have a semi-crystalloid structure and are inflammatory particles that induce an acute inflammatory response. As with crystals, the initial acute inflammation is self-limiting, but a subsequent chronic, foreign body granulomatous response shortly ensues and persists until the plant material is removed.

Plant-thorn synovitis and tenosynovitis mainly occur in children during play or in adults during fruit-picking or gardening. The hand and knee are most commonly affected and monoarticular presentation is usual. The injury may occur days before symptoms develop and is therefore often forgotten. The usual presumptive diagnosis of sepsis is often reinforced as the acute attack settles with antibiotics. Recurrence of persistent synovitis, however, requires consideration of other causes of monoarthritis, for example:
• chronic infection (including mycobacteria)
• initial presentation of juvenile chronic arthritis
• malignancy
• pigmented villonodular synovitis
• sarcoidosis (adults)

Radiographs may just show soft tissue swelling, or, less commonly, erosive cystic change; periosteal reaction is occasionally marked producing malignant-looking layered periostitis. Lesions appear hot on bone scans and the ESR is often elevated. Synovial fluid is usually inflammatory (low viscosity, turbid, increased cells, predominantly polymorphs); polarised microscopy of a spun pellet may rarely reveal birefringent plant material. The diagnosis is usually only confirmed following synovectomy. All plant material must be removed if the lesion is to resolve.

Occasionally atypical mycobacteria or other organisms travel in with the thorn and produce secondary infection. The black thorn (prunus spinosus) is the usual culprit, producing problems mainly in late summer and autumn. In adults rose thorns are equally common. A similar clinical picture may occur from the sun-dried tips of fallen palm fronds or following penetration by sea-urchin spines (these are predominately crystalline calcite).

34 (a) Linear radiolucencies, perpendicular to the surface, with associated sclerosis on the medial aspect of the upper femur (Looser's zone, "pseudo-fracture").
(b) Osteomalacia.
(c) Chronic anticonvulsant drug therapy and/or nutritional deficiency (ethnic).

In osteomalacia (soft bones) there is failure of bone mineralisation resulting histologically in excess of poorly calcified osteoid. In children (rickets) there is additional defective cartilage mineralisation, particularly epiphyseal growth plates. It most commonly results from vitamin D deficiency. The full clinical syndrome in adults comprises:
• diffuse bone pain and tenderness (especially ribs, spine, femora)
• fracture (commonly ribs)
• proximal muscle weakness (+/- wasting, hypotonia); waddling, Trendelenburg gait.
  It is uncommon for all features to be present, especially in the elderly. A high degree of suspicion is therefore required. Radiographs may show non-specific generalised osteopenia with cortical thinning; Looser's zones are characteristic but uncommon. In contrast to stress fractures (the principal differential diagnosis) Looser's zones are commonly painless, do not extend through both cortices and have no associated callus formation. They are often symmetrical targeting ribs, long bones (especially inner proximal femora), lateral scapulae and pelvic rami. The commonest biochemical abnormality is a raised alkaline phosphatase; serum calcium and phosphate may be low (25-hydroxyvitamin D and 1,25-dihydroxyvitamin D estimations are not generally available). Bone biopsy (following tetracycline labelling) provides the gold standard and ideally should be undertaken in all suspected cases; the combination of increased osteoid and reduced mineralisation is characteristic.
  Important causes of vitamin D deficiency are lack of sunlight, poor nutrition and malabsorption. Several risk factors often coexist (particularly in elderly subjects) and the Asian community is particularly at risk. Less common causes of osteomalacia include:
• **impaired hydroxylation of vitamin D to active metabolites**
  chronic renal failure; tumour-induced; hepatic osteodystrophy; vitamin D dependency rickets Type I
• **end organ resistance to 1,25 dihydroxyvitamin D**
  vitamin D dependency rickets Type II
• **hypophosphataemic states**
  inherited hypophosphataemia; Fanconi syndrome; tumour-induced
• **bone poisons**
  aluminium; bisphosphonates; fluoride
• **miscellaneous**
  chronic metabolic acidosis; chronic haemodialysis; chronic parenteral nutrition
  "Anticonvulsant osteomalacia" (resulting from increased turnover of 25-hydroxyvitamin D secondary to hepatic microsomal enzyme induction or effects on intestinal calcium absorption – mainly phenytoin)

Nutritional osteomalacia is treated by replacement of Vitamin D. A diagnostic trial of vitamin D (without biopsy) is often undertaken if for any reason bone biopsy proves problematic.

35 (a) Particulate semi-crystalline steroid.
(b) Steroid-induced synovitis and facial flushing.

Complications of local steroid injection include:
• skin and fat atrophy/telangiectasia/scarring (particularly with fluorinated steroids)
• facial flushing
• sepsis
• exacerbation of synovitis (microcrystalline depot steroid)
• tendon rupture if intratendinous injection given
• temporary exacerbation of diabetes
Although steroid-induced facial flushing is short-lived (36–48 hours) it is common (c.20% intra-articular injections) and may cause discomfort and distress, particularly if the patient has not been warned of its possibility.
Exacerbation of synovitis is uncommon and relates to the microcrystalline nature of some long-acting steroid preparations. Such exacerbation is generally mild and self-limiting over a few days and requires no specific treatment other than aspiration. The possibility of iatrogenic sepsis should always be excluded. Particulate steroid may remain detectable in synovial fluid for several weeks following injection. Such crystals are variable in shape and size (usually small rods c.1–8um), show no regular geometric form, may be intra- or extra-cellular, and display weak (positive or negative) birefringence. They may cause diagnostic confusion with other crystals.

36 (a) Henoch Schonlein purpura (HSP).
(b) Mild, transient synovitis usually involving a few large joints (commonly knees, ankles); chronic damage/deformity do not result. Myalgia or painful swelling of muscle or fascial tissue are uncommon.

HSP is common in children (mainly aged four to 11) but may occur at any age. It is characterised by:
• erythematous/purpuric rash (palpable)
• arthritis
• haematuria (glomerulonephritis)
• colicky abdominal pain (angio-oedema)
Oedema of lower legs is also common; occasionally oedema is periorbital, or affects hands, scalp, and perineum. Triggers include viral/bacterial infections, food allergy, and drugs but most cases are idiopathic. Biopsy of the skin and gut reveals leucocytoclastic vasculitis of small vessels (especially post-capillary venules). A characteristic finding is IgA deposition in skin and renal mesangium (similar to IgA nephropathy (Berger's disease)); IgA complexes may be detectable in serum but serum complement levels (and degradation products) are typically normal.
Most children recover uneventfully within three to four weeks. A minority follow a chronic or relapsing course. The overall prognosis relates to the

degree of renal involvement and nephrotic syndrome; severe and permanent renal damage is uncommon. Treatment is mainly supportive. NSAIDs or salicylate help joint symptoms; a short course of steroids is indicated for severe disease.

37 (a) He has a central lesion above the level of C4 but below the brain-stem.
(b) Abnormal (increased) movement between posterior arch of atlas and anterior aspect of the odontoid peg.
(c) Upper cervical cord compression/dysfunction due to atlanto-axial insta-bility

The usual causes of atlantoaxial subluxation are:
• RA (adult or juvenile-onset)
• ankylosing spondylitis (rare)
• severe neck trauma
    It can damage C2 nerve roots, vertebral arteries, upper cervical cord or brainstem. In RA it generally occurs as a late complication in patients with severe peripheral joint damage, especially following steroid treatment. Quadraplegia or sudden death may result. More typically, however, onset is insidious with symptoms confined to hands or feet. The patient often emphasises altered function more than sensation, particularly:
• clumsiness or weakness of one or both hands
• weakness, difficulty with walking ("going off my feet")
• altered sphincter control
    Neck/occipital pain is common and often severe. Neurological signs are often subtle and may be difficult to elicit or interpret due to spinal vessel damage (extending cord dysfunction to other levels), joint damage and peripheral neuropathy. Useful reflexes in this situation are:
• pectoralis jerk: present in upper motor lesions above C4
• jaw jerk: if normal the lesion is below the brainstem
• corneal reflex: often reduced in high cervical cord lesions (the sensory division of cranial nerve V is inversely represented in the upper cervical spine)
    A high level of clinical suspicion, and low threshold for investigation, are therefore necessary. Plain radiographs (AP, lateral extension and flexion, through-the-mouth odontoid views) usually clearly show:
• anterior, posterior or lateral antlantoaxial subluxation
• atlantoaxial impaction (cranial settling)
• subaxial subluxation
    However, radiographic abnormality only loosely correlates with neuro-logical involvement and MRI or CT studies are required to delineate the level and nature of the lesion. Indications for surgery include intractable pain and neurological involvement (myelopathy or radiculopathy).
    This patient had a single level of cord compression with no major sub-axial structural change. After a period in halo traction (to reduce deformity and improve neurological function) he underwent successful surgical fusion.

38 (a) Prepatellar bursitis.
(b) Aspiration: symptomatic drugs (analgesics, NSAIDs) if required; avoid-ance of or protection against provoking trauma.

The swelling (a) appears smooth, well circumscribed, and anterior to the patella; it shows no erythema and does not appear tense. On inspection alone, chronic prepatellar bursitis is the likely diagnosis. Palpation confirmed localised tenderness and a balloon sign (fluctuance) as the only regional abnormality. Detailed enquiry into his occupation confirmed repetitive kneeling on hard surfaces with no appropriate knee padding.

Three bursae around the patella commonly cause symptoms:
• prepatellar bursitis (as in this man)
• superficial infra-patellar bursitis, producing localised swelling readily visible below the patella anterior to the patellar tendon
• deep infra-patellar bursitis, producing less prominent swelling either side of the patellar tendon (similar to a large infrapatellar fat pad)

All three may be locally tender to palpation, feel warm, and show a balloon sign (pressure over one part of the swelling causes palpable bulging at the other anatomical boundaries).

Bursitis around the patella may arise from:
• occupational/recreational trauma (most common)
• sepsis
• systemic inflammatory disease (eg rheumatoid)
• crystal synovitis (gout, calcific periarthritis)
• foreign body reaction (eg plant-thorn synovitis)
• tumour (eg pigmented villonodular synovitis)

Carpet fitting, tiling, plumbing, mining, building and other physically exacting occupations particularly predispose to peripatellar bursitis, and these common traumatic lesions predominate in men. The old terms "housemaids" (prepatellar) and "clergyman's" (superficial infrapatellar) bursitis are thus increasingly inappropriate.

Appropriate management, as with most periarticular lesions, hinges upon identification of the cause via thorough history and examination. Examination of the bursal aspirate is required for diagnosis of sepsis and gout; recurrent blood-stained aspirates suggest pigmented villonodular synovitis and requirement for biopsy/excision. Plain radiographs will show calcific deposits (rare). Aspiration and analgesics/NSAIDs may temporarily alleviate symptoms and steroid injection may confer even greater short-term benefit. Avoidance of unnecessary trauma, or appropriate protection during occupational trauma, is essential if this appears causal. Control of underlying rheumatoid disease or gout by appropriate drug therapy is often curative.

39 (a) Nodal generalized osteoarthritis (NGOA) with Heberden's and Bouchard's nodes.
(b) Hypoplasia of the hand with small muscle wasting.
(c) The sparing effect of a neurological deficit (in this case a lower motor neurone lesion due to childhood poliomyelitis) on subsequent development of arthritis.

This woman's history is typical of NGOA. It usually presents in women around the menopause ("menopausal arthritis") as a stuttering-onset polyarthritis of DIPJs and PIPJs. Symptoms occur while posterolateral Heberden's and Bouchard's nodes and associated interphalangeal OA are developing. However, once the nodes are fully evolved symptoms slowly abate. The outcome with respect to symptoms and hand function is generally excellent. The term "generalised" is included because such patients are at increased risk of subsequent development of bilateral knee and/or hip OA (as in this case). There is strong familial predisposition to NGOA, and a putative association with HLA A1B8.

Hypoplasia of one hand with motor but not sensory deficit is consistent with childhood polio. Both upper and lower motor neurone lesions may protect against subsequent development of arthropathy on the paretic side. This has been reported for RA, gout, NGOA and psoriatic arthritis. Conversely if development of arthritis precedes an acute neurological deficit exacerbation of arthritis may be triggered within a few weeks on the paretic side. Such ipsilateral acute exacerbation has been reported for RA and rapidly destructive (apatite-associated) OA. The mechanism(s) related to sparing or triggering of arthropathy by neurological lesions is ill-understood.

Other aetiological associations of interest include (a) triggering of ipsilateral reflex sympathetic dystrophy syndrome by acute neurological deficit, and (b) production of neuropathic arthropathy by a chronic neurological deficit.

40 (a) Soft tissue swelling, marginal erosions, and cartilage loss mainly affecting second and fifth MTPJs and big toe IPJ; osseous cysts big toe IPJ; hallux valgus.
(b) RA.

The forefoot is very commonly involved in RA and is often the first site in the patient (even if asymptomatic) to show radiographic erosions. Individual radiographic features of RA include:
• soft-tissue swelling (synovitis, bursitis, tenosynovitis, tendinitis, nodules)
• osteopenia (juxta-articular; later generalised)
• marginal non-proliferative erosion (occurring first at "bare" areas close to synovial/capsular insertions)
• joint space narrowing (usually late, pancompartmental)
• osseous cysts
• deformity, subluxation, (late)
• ankylosis (occasional at wrist and midfoot)
• stress fracture (late, particularly lower tibia/fibula)

Target sites in the forefoot are MTPJs. Early erosions predominate on the metatarsal side, mainly the medial aspect of the first to fourth metatarsal heads and lateral and medial aspects of the fifth (a); earliest erosions often affect the first or fifth. The big toe IPJ is commonly affected, the most extensive lesion predominating on the medial aspect of the proximal phalanx. Severe involvement of this joint is uncommon (cf. seronegative spondarthritis). As the disease progresses typical deformities include:
• hallux valgus
• lateral (fibular) deviation at first-fourth MTPJs
• medial (tibial) deviation at fifth MTPJ
• "cock-up" toes (hyperextension of MTPJs with dorsal subluxation of proximal phalanges, plantar subluxation of metatarsal heads, secondary IPJ flexion)

41 (a) Lupus pernio.
(b) Asymmetrical soft tissue swelling; marked erosion, expansion and deformity of distal phalanges; cartilage loss with destruction of articular cortex

(NB retained bone density).
(c) Chronic sarcoidosis.

Acute sarcoid is common, often presents with erythema nodosum or symptomatic thoracic involvement (with radiographic hilar lymphadenopathy), and usually undergoes spontaneous resolution without sequelae. Chronic sarcoid, however, is rare, mainly affects older, middle-aged subjects (women more than men) and may cause joint damage and disability.

Mono- or oligo-arthritis involving knees or ankles is most common, though symmetrical small and large joint arthropathy may simulate RA. Osseous involvement particularly targets small bones of feet and hands (rarely skull, vertebrae, long bones). Granulomatous infiltration causes cystic lesions, cortical erosion and bone resorption with adjacent soft-tissue "spongy" swelling but retained bone density. Although uncommon, cortical thickening with fine "lacy" reticular alteration of trabecular pattern is characteristic. Other uncommon locomotor manifestations include tenosynovitis and carpal tunnel syndrome. Muscle involvement is common but usually asymptomatic. Although sarcoidosis is a multisystem disease, bone and joint involvement particularly associate with:

• skin involvement: raised violaceous skin plaques (in this patient occurring over face and nose as classic lupus pernio) or keloids
• parenchymal lung disease (fibrosis +/- cor-pulmonale)

Skin lesions and an abnormal chest x-ray are therefore usually present to suggest the diagnosis. Over 50% of patients also have concomitant eye involvement (mainly iritis +/- secondary glaucoma; less commonly chorioretinitis, keratoconjunctivitis sicca). Other, less common, clinical features include lymphadenopathy, hepatosplenomegaly, cranial nerve palsy, hypopituitarism, peripheral polyneuropathy, pericarditis and arrythmias.

The diagnosis is usually suggested by recognition of multisystem involvement with typical changes on chest and joint radiographs. If tissue confirmation is required typical sarcoid granulomata may be obtained from biopsy of synovium or skin. "Blind" needle muscle biopsy is also often positive. Although the Kveim-Siltzbach test is positive in most patients with acute sarcoidosis, it may be negative in chronic disease.

Management is mainly symptomatic (local physical therapy, analgesics, NSAIDs). Steroids are commonly tried but the response is often disappointing. The case for hydroxychloroquine or cytotoxic therapy remains unproven. This patient experienced improvement in joint symptoms and malaise with low-dose steroid and azathioprine – her lupus pernio, however, remained unchanged.

42 (a) Chronic iritis (anterior uveitis) producing an irregular right pupil due to synechiae.
(b) Chronic erosive enthesopathy with extensive new-bone proliferation at the Achilles tendon and plantar fascia insertions.
(c) Chronic Reiter's disease.

Ocular manifestations of Reiter's disease include conjunctivitis, uveitis, or keratitis. Conjunctivitis is a common early manifestation; often bilateral, symptoms of pain, burning, or itching usually last days rather than weeks. Uveitis is usually acute, unilateral, and unassociated with chorioretinitis; it complicates established disease and may be chronic or relapsing. If untreated it may seriously compromise vision. Uveitis is a frequent extra-articular feature of seronegative spondyloarthropathy, especially in classic ankylosing spondylitis (c.30%). Lone uveitis is not uncommon in the community and associates with HLA B27 even in the absence of spondarthritis (pelvis x-ray for occult sacroiliitis is a standard screen).

Psoriatic arthropathy and chronic Reiter's show considerable overlap (eg asymmetric arthropathy, nail dystrophy, skin lesions, spondylitis with coarse non-marginal syndesmophytes, and asymmetric sacroiliitis). However, unlike psoriasis, hand involvement is rare in Reiter's, and typical psoriatic plaques are absent (NB keratoderma blenorrhagica is identical to pustular psoriasis); conversely, chronic iritis is uncommon with psoriasis. Calcaneal enthesopathy, particulary at the plantar aponeurosis and long plantar ligament origins, is common in both. In Reiter's it is usually unilateral and occurs early. Enthesitis (inflammation at fibrous insertions into periosteum or bone) initially erodes bone but then stimulates exuberant repair with fluffy new bone formation. Such ossifying enthesopathy is often more prominent than the "spurs" seen in other seronegative or inflammatory arthritis (eg RA), and contrasts with the smaller, smoother, non-erosive spurs associated with traumatic/degenerative change. Diffuse idiopathic skeletal hyperostosis is the other principal cause of exuberant entheseal bone proliferation.

43 (a) Palatal ulceration with surrounding erythema.
(b) High swinging pyrexia peaking in the evening with associated tachycardia.
(c) Systemic onset juvenile chronic arthritis (Still's Disease).

This condition is usually seen in infants or young children, girls more than boys. It usually begins abruptly with malaise and high remitting fever. Around 50% patients have an evanescent, usually pruritic, maculopapular salmon pink eruption mainly on the trunk (but also over joints, palms and soles), most marked during febrile episodes or after a hot bath. Sore throat and mucosal lesions (as in this patient) are common. Inflammatory joint involvement is usual but may occur late or be overlooked; it is usually symmetrical, targeting knees, wrists and cervical spine (CS). Serositis may result in symptoms of pericarditis, pleurisy and abdominal pain. Lymphadenopathy occurs in most cases, splenomegaly less often. Subcutaneous nodules are rare and histologically resemble those of rheumatic fever rather than RA. Eye involvement is predominately iritis though band keratopathy (opacities in the cornea) and glaucoma and cataract (late) may occur. All children with Still's disease need screening by an opthalmologist using slit-lamp examination.

Investigations usually reveal moderate or severe anaemia, a marked leukocytosis (neutrophilia) and florid acute phase response. Immunoglobulins show polyclonal increase; autoantibodies (including IgM rheumatoid factor) are usually negative and complement activation is uncommon. The diagnosis is essentially clinical and one of exclusion. Sepsis and malignancy are often considered first and certainly need investigation. Early joint x-rays may show periarticular osteoporosis and periostitis; erosions are rare and principal late features are chondropathy with subsequent ankylosis and growth defects (especially carpometacarpal joints and cervical spine).

Treatment, best accomplished with a multi-disciplinary team, aims to control pain, prevent loss and to restore range of joint movement, minimise/control inflammation and ensure normal physical and psychological growth. NSAIDs are the first line of drug treatment; high-dose aspirin has now been replaced by other NSAIDs which are given at higher dose/weight than adults (because of efficient hepatic function). In severe disease second-line drugs are used, the best evidence being for methotrexate (though hydroxychloroquine, sulphasalazine and gold are still often tried). Steroids are used for severe systemic upset, particularly with serositis; they are given for short periods, often using alternate-day single dosage schedules to reduce growth disturbances. Intra-articualr steroids for troublesome joints are extremely useful. Physiotherapy plays an important role in acute and long-term management of these patients. Surgery may be neccesary in severe cases with limiting deformities.

44 (a) Lumbar myelogram demonstrating abscess formation with cord compression. Loss of cortex and osseous destruction of fourth and fifth vertebra (particularly anteriorly); obliteration of L4/L5 disc space; minor vertebral osteophyte and intervertebral narrowing at higher levels.
(b) Pyogenic osteomyelitis (*Staphylococcus aureus*) complicating his urogential procedure.

The pathological and clinical features of infections involving vertebral bodies and discs are conditioned by anatomy, principally the blood supply. The arterial supply follows the embryological pattern: one intercostal artery supplies two vertebrae (the lower half of one and the upper half of the vertebra below) and a rich anastamosis of vessels around the posterior aspect of the bodies penetrate anteriorly to anastamose with segmental structures. Infections thus tend to involve the adjacent parts of two vertebrae and intervening cartilaginous disc, localising in the cartilaginous end plate because of specialised vascular tufts in this area. Most infections arrive in arterial blood though venous-spread infection also occurs. An important predisposing factor is genitourinary instrumentation (as in this patient) because of the connection between the pelvic and vetebral venous plexus of Batson.

S. aureus is the commonest causative organism; others include pseudomonas, *E. Coli*, salmonella, typhoid and brucella. Two-thirds of infections involve the lumbar spine, vertebral bodies being targeted more than the posterior neural arch. The initial focus in or around the vertebral end plate spreads to involve adjacent cancellous bone and disc; necrosis of both then results from impaired blood supply (especially to the disc) and inflammatory destruction. Bony collapse results in progressive anterior vertebral wedging and obliteration of disc space. Abscess formation is common but generally less marked than with TB; initially paravertebral, it may track in various directions depending on the level involved. Spinal cord compression, resulting in paraplegia, is relatively uncommon in pyogenic (cf. tuberculous) infection. More typically there is new bone formation anteriorly and laterally with tendency to fusion of adjacent bodies. In many cases, especially in the elderly, the disease runs a mild course, the only changes being narrowing of the disc space and reactive sclerosis of adjacent bodies.

Broadly two patterns of presentation are seen. Firstly, acute onset with severe constitutional upset, high fever, localised back pain and severe nerve root pain, with marked muscle spasm and restriction of movement. Secondly (most common), insidious onset over weeks or months of intermittent back pain and mild constitutional upset; muscle spasm and restriction of movement are minimal or absent. Radiographic changes are slow to appear and lag behind clinical features by one to two months. Isotope bone scans and MRI are both far more sensitive. Other appropriate investigations include ESR, CRP, blood cultures, bacterial titres and a tuberculin test. The organism in this patient was *S. aureus* (isolated from blood cultures). His abscess was aspirated and decompressed surgically, and he made an excellent recovery following an initial period of rest and parenteral antibiotics (continued orally for six weeks).

45 (a) Monosodium urate crystals (compensated polarised light microscopy).
(b) Tophaceous gout and chronic Reiter's disease.

There is natural reluctance to make two diagnoses in the same system in a patient. This man had chronic Reiter's disease with confirmed spondylitis. However, his peripheral arthropathy sounded atypical for this. For example:
- though chronic Reiter's can affect lower limb joints (classically hindfoot, knee or hip) with chronic mono- or oligoarthritis, relapsing acute episodes are unusual
- in the big toe the interphalangeal, not first MTPJ, is the usual target joint.
- chronic Reiter's (unlike radiographically identical psoriatic spondylitis) uncommonly affects upper limb joints
- nodules are not a feature
  Conditions that cause both arthritis and nodules include:
- RA
- gout (tophi)
- hyperlipidaemia (xanthomata)
- rheumatic fever (small nodules)
- lupus (small nodules)
- multicentric reticulohistiocytosis
- polyarteritis nodosa
  In the first five conditions nodules predominate at similar sites over bony extensor surfaces (wrists, elbows, knees, heels). Rheumatoid nodules inevitably associate with seropositivity, so other causes needed consideration in this man.

The classic progression of untreated male gout is from recurrent attacks in lower limb joints (including podagra in first MTPJs) to chronic tophaceous gout involving distal upper limb, and more proximal lower limb, joints. Gout would therefore seem the likely second diagnosis in this man.

Confirmation of gout is by identification of monosodium urate monohydrate (MSUM) crystals, usually in synovial fluid or tophus aspirate. If seen during an intercritical period the diagnosis can be confirmed on synovial fluid aspirated from an asymptomatic knee or first metatarsophalangeal joint. MSUM crystals are needle shaped (c.4–20u long), show strong (negative) birefringence (Figure *b*), and are soluble in uricase. They are mainly intracellular during attacks, and extracellular between attacks. In tophi they occur as dense parallel sheets (Figure *c*). Serum uric acid levels are unreliable for diagnosis; a high level does not confirm gout (hyperuricaemia is more common than gout) and normal or low levels do not exclude the diagnosis.

The associations of "primary" gout include:
- obesity
- excessive alcohol consumption
- hyperlipidaemia (c.30%)
- hypertension
- urate nephropathy and uric acid nephrolithiasis
  "Secondary" gout may relate to:
- chronic diuretic therapy
- chronic renal impairment
- lead poisoning (seen in "moonshine" drinkers; lead used to be added to port as a sweetener, explaining the old association with port)

Very high serum levels of uric acid may occur with cytotoxic therapy for malignancy and in acute renal failure. However, this results in renal rather than joint problems (urate crystals usually take months or years to deposit and grow in locomotor tissues).

This patient had primary gout with no apparent risk factors. He was treated with allopurinol to maintain his uric acid in the lower half of the normal range. After two years his tophi had regressed and he was suffering no further flares of arthritis.

46 (a) Ulnar deviation and subluxation of MCPJs; swan-neck deformities; some cartilage loss (mainly radiocarpal, carpometacarpal joints); possible minor erosive change (IPJs).
(b) SLE.

This patient's radiograph shows predominantly non-erosive deformity atypical of long-standing RA but characteristic of arthritis in SLE. Her other symptoms and seropositivity for rheumatoid factor are also consistent with a diagnosis of SLE.

Joint involvement is the most frequent manifestation of SLE. Arthralgia and stiffness affect >95% of patients at some time, and objective signs (eg stress pain, effusion, tenosynovitis) are present in the majority at time of diagnosis (tenosynovitis is often more prominent than synovitis). Joint symptoms may precede multisystem disease by many years. Involvement is usually symmetrical and principally targets IPJs, knees, wrists and MCPJs. Non-erosive deforming arthritis occurs in c.10% of patients and may rarely associate with small rheumatoid nodules. Joint deformities, as in this case, result from chronic inflammation and weakening mainly of periarticular structures (tendons, ligaments) and joint capsules with little cartilage or bone attrition. SLE patients are also more prone to joint sepsis and avascular necrosis which may require consideration and exclusion. Avascular necrosis typically affects hips, though knees, elbows, shoulders and carpal bones may also be affected (mainly in those who have received steroids). Non-specific myalgia is common in those with active disease, especially with lymphocytic vasculitis; polymyositis may occur in overlap syndromes.

It should also be recognised that patients with SLE may, in common with the normal population, suffer non-associated conditions (eg osteoarthritis, mechanical back pain, fibromyalgia) and careful clinical assessment is always required before attributing locomotor symptoms to active disease.

47 (a) Flexor tenosynovitis.
(b) Triggering; rupture.
(c) Trauma (most common); gout; disseminated gonococcal arthritis (DGI); enteropathic arthritis.

Flexor tenosynovitis, and associated tendinitis, are common in RA. It is readily felt as a linear, soft tissue swelling in the palm, often tender, with crepitus on active/passive finger movement. Swelling is most usual over the second/third tendons. Swelling and crepitus may also occur at the distal forearm immediately proximal to the wrist creases, and along the volar aspect of fingers between the tight skin creases. Tight power grip is made difficult and fingers feel stiff/tight, particularly in the morning; true triggering is unusual unless complicated by intra-tendinous rheumatoid nodules. If marked, a fixed flexion attitude is usual. Tendon rupture may result (especially with intratendinous nodules), usually at the MCPJ level as the tendons enter the finger; the third flexor tendon is most commonly affected followed by the second, fourth, fifth and first. Trauma-related tenosynovitis affects fewer tendons, most commonly the first (thumb). It often relates to repetitive manual work and improves if such trauma is avoided. Stenosing tenovaginitis is fibrous constriction of the tendon sheath; this causes pressure/friction effects on the tendon especially where it passes through tight encasing rings/pulleys partly comprise an osseous groove (eg flexor surface of metacarpal). The tendon enlarges distal to the constriction, resulting in a snapping sensation (triggering) as the swelling has to negotiate the narrowed segment. Locking in flexion occurs when the flexor muscle, but not the relatively weaker extensor, can overcome this obstruction; forced extension may permit "unlocking".

Concurrence of tenosynovitis and dermatitis should suggest DGI; tenosynovitis (especially bilateral) rarely accompanies other causes of septic arthritis. Multiple tendons are usually involved simultaneously, especially around wrists, fingers, ankles and toes. Tenosynovitis of fingers or toes may occur in enteropathic arthritis and in chronic gout. Wrist flexor tenosynovitis is an occasional feature of hypothyrodism and diabetes.

Treatment is usually conservative (rest, temporary splinting, analgesia, local corticosteroid injection) with surgery reserved for resistant cases. Usual sites for stenosing tenosynovitis are the thumb flexor/extensor, finger flexors, flexor carpi radialis (pain at proximal thenar eminence), common peroneal sheath (pain below/behind lateral malleolus), tibialis posterior tendon (pain below/behind medial malleolus after prolonged walking and standing).

48 (a) Knee OA.
(b) Obesity, degree of varus deformity and being female are poor risk factors for progression. Other suggested factors include poor quadriceps tone, instability, presence of effusions, associated chondrocalcinosis, and chronic NSAID ingestion.

The knee is a common target site for OA. Involvement is often bilateral, particularly in women and in the elderly. Although it may occur as a mono- or pauci-articular problem (particularly in men) this site shows strong association with hand OA. The medial tibiofemoral and patellofemoral compartments are particularly involved, severe attrition of the medial compartment giving the characteristic varus deformity, best assessed during weight-bearing (Figure *a*).

This man's standard (non weight-bearing) AP x-ray shows osteophyte in both compartments, and sclerosis with altered bone contour and joint space loss in the medial compartment. The extreme degree of cartilage loss, however, is only apparent on the standing view when the two opposing bony surfaces fit together (standing films should be used to assess tibiofemoral OA).

Risk factors for development of knee OA include:
• obesity
• being female
• trauma (eg previous meniscectomy)
• generalised OA
• distal femoral dysplasia
(NB smoking appears to have a negative association)

Obesity and being female are probably the two most important risk factors both for development and progression. Successful correction of obesity has now been shown to improve symptomatic outcome. In addition to increased morbidity, knee OA associates with increased mortality (possibly due to NSAIDs).

This man's symptoms continued to progress despite quadriceps exercises and symptomatic measures and he underwent successful total knee replacements one year later.

49 (a) Marginal/subchondral erosions, apparent widening of joint space, subluxations, and soft tissue swelling, predominating in interphalangeal and first carpometacarpal joints.
(b) Multicentric reticulohistiocytosis (MRH).
(c) Histological demonstration of multinucleate giant cells and histiocytes with granular "foamy" cytoplasm containing lipoid material (staining positively with PAS and Sudan black). Biopsy material is usually taken from skin nodules or synovium, but may also be positive from muscle, liver and other tissues.

MRH is a rare disease characterised by destructive polyarthritis and nodular skin lesions. It predominates in middle-aged women. Symmetrical polyarthritis of small and large joints often precedes skin lesions by months or years. Weight loss and general malaise may be prominent. Routine investigations show only a mild acute phase response and it is inevitably misdiagnosed as RA until skin lesions or distinctive radiographic changes appear. The chronic skin lesions are small yellow or purplish nodules which particularly locate around nailfolds, dorsum of hands, forearms, ears, nose and neck. Disfiguring infiltrative swelling of skin also occurs (as in this patient's fingers (Figure *a*) and may produce a "leonine" facies. Arthritis causes pain, stiffness, swelling and tenderness; severe destruction and instability (arthritis "mutilans") often occurs within a few years. Radiographs show erosive change, but features which may permit distinction from RA (well shown in Figure *b*) include:

- erosions across the end plate
- widening, rather than loss of joint space
- predominance of interphalangeal joint involvement
- relatively retained bone density

The cause remains unclear. Although xanthelesmata and hyperlipoproteinaemia occur in up to 30% of patients there is no evidence of a primary metabolic abnormality; the lipid accumulation in infiltrating giant cells and histiocytes appears non-specific. Various malignancies have been reported to develop in up to 30% of cases.

There is no treatment of proven efficacy though cytotoxics have particularly been advocated. Spontaneous remissions may occur, but often only after destructive arthritis is established. The skin lesions, joint symptoms and malaise in this patient were greatly improved by use of cyclophosphamide. Unfortunately haemorrhagic cystitis required cessation of cyclophosphamide and within two months the nodules and joint symptoms reappeared. A second remission appeared to follow use of azathioprine.

50 (a) Bilateral shoulder effusions with extensive subacromial/subdeltoid extension (left) and anterior pectoral extension (right); muscle wasting (particularly evident on the right).
(b) RA.

The shoulder joint and peri-articular tissues are commonly involved in both early and late RA. Subacromial bursitis causes lateral pain with radiation down the upper arm, especially if communicating with the large subdeltoid bursa. There may be swelling and a painful middle arc. Rotator cuff tendinitis (+/- partial or complete tears) causes upper arm pain, reproduced by resisted active movement; a painful middle arc occurs with supraspinatus lesions and passive abduction is usually full (cf glenohumeral arthritis). Bicipital tendinitis causes anterior upper arm pain reproduced by resisted active wrist supination or elbow flexion (elbow held in mid-flexion); local tenderness in the bicipital groove (between greater and lesser tuberosities) is usual. Chronic inflammation may result in bicipital tendon rupture.

Acromioclavicular joint involvement causes localised pain and tenderness (+/- swelling) over the joint. Night pain when lying on the affected side is common; a superior painful arc (last 15°) is usual and pain is reproduced by forced adduction or raising the humerus against a fixed clavicle. Glenohumeral arthropathy causes upper arm pain (deriving from C5 embryonic segment). Abduction and external rotation are initially painful but eventually all movements are restricted. Global wasting occurs in established disease. Effusions usually present anteriorly medial to the coracoid process though coexistent rotator cuff damage will permit fluid to distend the subacromial and subdeltoid bursae (as in this patient). Active and passive movements are equally restricted and there is anterior joint line tenderness. Osteonecrosis of the humeral head may occur spontaneously (rare) or complicate systemic steroid therapy. Involvement of the sternoclavicular joint causes local swelling and tenderness and pain on elevating the arm.

Chronic effusions may result in thick, inspissated fluid, sometimes containing cholesterol crystals, which is poorly cleared by compromised lymphatics. This may result in florid capsular and bursal extensions which track into low-resistance tissue planes, as in this patient. Fluid is often loculated and difficult to aspirate. Sinus formation may complicate this picture ("fistulous rheumatoid").

51 (a) SLE (with renal involvement).
(b) Steroid (limited early treatment) with cytotoxic (cyclophosphamide, azathioprine or methotrexate) continued as principal treatment.

Photosensitivity occurs in c.30% of SLE patients. Sun (ultraviolet light) exposure has been implicated as a cause of disease exacerbation in SLE and may account for reported seasonal variations in disease activity and incidence. Direct sunshine is not required since the responsible UV light can penetrate cloud cover. The classic butterfly rash occurs on both cheeks and across the bridge of the nose and is usually considered as sunburn by most patients; it usually heals well with no scarring. Differentiation is from seborrhoeic dermatitis (this targets nasolabial folds which are spared in SLE) and acne rosacea (characterised by papules/pustules which are not a feature of SLE unless secondary infection is present). Biopsy (rarely indicated) shows epidermal thinning, liquefaction of basal epidermis, disruption of dermal-epidermal junction, and dermal oedema with scattered lymphocytic infiltrates particularly around upper dermal capillaries. Mucosal ulceration is also common in SLE (c.40%), often affecting the hard or soft palate (less commonly nasal septum) and usually, though not always, being symptomatic. Such ulceration usually accompanies active disease flares.

Lupus nephritis may present with any renal syndrome and used to be the major cause of death from lupus. It is relatively unusual as the initial manifestation but is more common in children and young adults with SLE. Any component of the kidney may be involved. Glomerular lesions range from mesangiopathy and focal proliferative glomerulonephritis (GN) to diffuse membranous GN and glomerulosclerosis. "Active" lesions include glomerular crescents, diffuse glomerular proliferation and interstitial mononuclear infiltrates; "chronic" lesions indicate scarring and comprise glomerular sclerosis and interstitial fibrosis. Renal vessels may be involved as part of a hypertensive or vasculitic process, and microthrombi in small vessels may associate with anticardiolipin antibodies. Because of this heterogeneity a low threshold for renal biopsy is appropriate for SLE patients with proteinuria and/or renal impairment; biopsy findings will guide the choice of treatment options designed to prevent deterioration of function. This patient had diffuse proliferative GN. He was initially given intravenous cyclophosphamide plus steroid; subsequent maintenance was with azathioprine and reducing prednisolone. Aspirin (+/- dipyridamole) is appropriate for patients with anticardiolipin antibodies and microthrombi; warfarin is an alternative. Careful follow-up, and treatment of coexistent hypertension, is indicated. This patient suffered no chronic renal impairment and did very well; he received cytotoxic treatment for two years. SLE is more common in females but males are not excluded; this patient had no congenital complement deficiency to explain his predisposition.

52 Ruptured long head of biceps.

Bicipital tendinitis is a common periarticular lesion usually resulting from mechanical overusage. It may occur in isolation but more commonly accompanies rotator cuff injury or glenohumeral instability. Pain is felt over the anterior shoulder and palpation reveals localised tenderness over the bicipital groove between greater and lesser tuberosities. The biceps is necessary for the "corkscrew" action for opening wine bottles (power wrist supination and elbow flexion) and pain of bicipital tendinitis is therefore reproduced by:
• resisted wrist supination with shoulder adducted and elbow at 90°
• resisted elbow flexion (starting at 90° flexion)
  Rupture of the tendon may occur spontaneously or follow steroid injection, as in this man. Rupture leads to impressive increase in muscle bulk on resisted active movements, but in the lower rather than middle third of the humerus (a). Rupture may occur at the glenoid labrum attachment or (with steroid-induced atrophy) as it runs in the bicipital groove.
  Bicipital tendinitis is treated by avoidance of provoking activities, physical therapy (including laser) and NSAIDs. Local steroid injection may quickly improve symptoms but care should be taken not to inject directly (felt as resistance) into the tendon. Failure to recognise and treat associated rotator cuff pathology or instability will lead to reccurrence. Tendon rupture is usually treated conservatively and for most activities, other than strenuous sport, results in surprisingly little functional impairment.

53 (a) Psoriasis.
(b) Scaly non-pruritic rash, classically on the extensor surfaces of the arms and legs; less obvious ("hidden") sites are the scalp, umbilicus, as in this case, and natal cleft. Nail lesions include pitting, ridging, discolouration, onycholysis and sub-ungal fibromata.
(c) Psoriasis associates with an increased prevalence of seronegative (psoriatic) arthropathy. The association is stronger for nail dystrophy than skin lesions.

Seronegative arthritis occurs in c.7% of psoriatic patients, representing a six- to ten-fold increase over non-psoriatic controls. A wide spectrum of axial and peripheral arthropathy may occur, but characteristic features of psoriatic arthropathy include:
• the pattern of involvement: "sausage digits" and asymmetrical large-joint lower-limb synovitis are common; inflammatory spondylitis, DIPJ predominant small-joint arthropathy, and inflammatory polyarthritis are less common.
• radiographic features: retained bone density, "proliferative" marginal erosions, periostitis, ossifying enthesopathy, and rarely marked bone resorption ("arthritis mutilans").
  When faced with an arthritis of unknown aetiology a careful search for skin and nail lesions is warranted. Skin lesions may precede, coincide with, or follow development of arthropathy. In the latter situation diagnosis is problematic unless the arthropathy is characteristic, eg sausage digit plus lower-limb (knee/ankle) synovitis). Nail pitting, however, often precedes clinically apparent skin lesions and is usually present in patients with psoriatic

arthropathy *sine* psoriasis. A family history of seronegative spondarthropathy may help support the diagnosis.

Although skin and joint symptoms may worsen in parallel, in most cases the activity and severity of psoriasis and arthropathy are dissociated, representing a disease association (as with inflammatory bowel disease and classic ankylosing spondylitis). It is noteworthy that psoriatic patients are not protected from development of other arthropathies – not all their problems will relate to psoriatic arthropathy.

54 (a) Red blood cells and polymorphs; weakly birefringent intracellular rods, typical of calcium pyrophosphate dihydrate (CPPD) crystals.
(b) Acute pseudogout.

The knee is the commonest target site for acute attacks of florid synovitis ("pseudogout") associated with CPPD crystal deposition. Pseudogout predominates in the elderly and may occur in previously asymptomatic knees or on a background of chronic arthritis showing clinical and radiographic features of osteoarthritis ("chronic pyrophosphate arthropathy"). Acute attacks involve "shedding" of CPPD crystals from preformed cartilage deposits. As with gout, shedding may be provoked by intercurrent events, most commonly local trauma, intercurrent illness or surgery. Haemarthrosis is not uncommon and principally reflects the florid nature of the acute inflammation. The principal differential diagnosis is gout or sepsis (all three may co-exist) and correct diagnosis requires synovial fluid examination and culture. Under compensated polarised microscopy CPPD crystals are short, thick, usually rhomboid rods (c.2–10um long), showing weak (positive) birefringence; they are mainly intracellular in acute attacks. Usually only small numbers are present and because of their size and weak birefringence they can easily be missed. Radiographic chondrocalcinosis is often, but not always, present to support the diagnosis.

Aspiration and simple analgesia usually suffice to settle the attack. NSAIDs, though often effective, are preferably avoided in the elderly, particularly in the presence of cardiac or renal impairment. Intra-articular steroid injection is useful for florid attacks, and successfully controlled the episode in this woman. Oral colchicine is also effective, though rarely required. Joint lavage is reserved for rare troublesome attacks resistant to other measures.

55 (a) Linear diaphyseal periostitis.
(b) Secondary hypertrophic osteoarthropathy (HOA).

HOA comprises:
• chronic proliferative periostitis of distal long (less commonly short) bones
• clubbing of fingers and toes
• oligo/polyarthritis: usually bilateral, symmetrical

Thickening and furrowing of facial skin ("leonine" facies), greasy skin and excess sweating are common additional features in primary HOA (pachydermoperiostitis). Primary HOA is rare, usually hereditary, predominates in men and presents around puberty; joint and periosteal symptoms are mild or absent. By contrast, in secondary HOA skin features are uncommon and locomotor symptoms predominate. Any cause of clubbing may

result in HOA, but lung causes (carcinoma, cystic fibrosis) are most common. The following causes of secondary HOA are recognised:
- pulmonary disease: benign or malignant neoplasm, bronchiectasis, abscess, empyema, fibrosing alveolitis
- cardiovascular: cyanotic congenital disease, bacterial endocarditis
- gastrointestinal: cirrhosis, inflammatory bowel disease, coeliac disease, malignancy (liver, colon, oesophagus)

Thyroid acropachy is the principal differential diagnosis. The onset may be acute (especially in malignancy) or insidious. Usually the underlying disease is apparent (as in this case), but HOA may precede manifestation of the causal disease by many months. Periostitis may cause severe, deep-seated burning pain of distal extremities. Characteristically the pain is worsened by dependency and improved by elevation. Joint symptoms vary from mild arthralgia to severe articular pain, particularly affecting MCPJs, wrists, elbows, knees and ankles. Distal extremities often appear broadened by firm, mildly pitting oedema. Distal long bones and affected joints are tender and warm and varying degrees of synovitis may be apparent. Gross clubbing is always apparent.

Early radiographs show proliferative, linear or irregular periostitis affecting the distal diaphysis and metaphysis of long bones and less commonly phalanges (Figure *b*). This new bone thickens and merges with the cortex as linear periostitis progresses proximally. Scintigraphy shows increased uptake before periostitis is apparent on plain films.

The pathogenesis is unknown, though increased vascularity secondary to neuronal reflexes, circulating hormones or immune complexes have been incriminated. Vagotomy and effective treatment of the underlying cause may result in resolution. Analgesics, NSAIDs, or steroids may help in incurable cases. This patient's symptoms were readily controlled by use of intermittent NSAIDs, injection of knees and wrists, and continuing aggressive treatment of his bronchiectasis.

56 (a) Giant, dilated nailfold capillary loops.
(b) Juvenile dermatomyositis.

An erythematous rash with raised, silvery-purple plaques (Gottron's papules) occurring over extensor surfaces of finger joints and elbows (often also knees, ankles) is typical of dermatomyositis; its appearance and distribution often mirrors psoriasis. Less common is the classic purplish ("heliotrope") rash on the eyelids and cheeks with periorbital oedema. Nailfold hyperaemia (evident in Figure *a*) is a common accompaniment. Individual large, dilated capillary loops may be visible by naked eye, but are more clearly seen using a dissecting microscope (after placing clear oil on the skin to prevent surface reflection). In other connective tissue diseases, including secondary Raynaud's that precedes other features, loss of loops and abnormal branching may be seen using this technique.

Unlike in adults, dermatomyositis in children and juveniles does not associate with malignancy. However, in children it may (a) be accompanied by systemic vasculitis, and (b) predispose to late atrophy and subcutaneous/perimyseal calcification.

In addition to proximal girdle muscle weakness this boy's neck flexors were weak, but he had no dysphagia or dysphonia to suggest bulbar muscle involvement. Respiratory function was normal (pulmonary fibrosis may occur, especially in those with anti Jo-1 antibodies). Bilateral, symmetrical arthralgia/mild synovitis in this distribution (+/- knees, elbows, shoulders) is common. His ESR was 88 and his creatine phosphokinase greatly elevated. Needle quadriceps biopsy confirmed dermatomyositis with no vasculitis. He responded well to oral prednisolone and weekly oral cyclophosphamide (12 doses). His rash and synovitis resolved within two weeks but, as is usual, objective muscle strength improved only after six weeks of treatment.

57 (a) DISH (diffuse idiopathic skeletal hyperostosis).
(b) Obesity, maturity-onset diabetes, ageing, hypervitaminosis A.

DISH (Forestier's disease, ankylosing hyperostosis) is a common condition in middle-aged and elderly caucasians (males more than females). It causes flowing, course "molten wax" ossification along the anterior and lateral aspects of the spine with bridging between vertebrae (Forestier''s disease). Any region may be involved though the thoracic spine is particularly targeted. In the upper thoracic region lesions are restricted to the right side, but elsewhere they are usually bilateral; in dextrocardia the left thoracic spine is involved, suggesting inhibition of abnormal new bone formation by the aortic pulsation. Lesions start at the ligamentous insertions away from the vertebral rim; bridging may be preceded by anterior ossifications close to the annulus fibres. In established lesions a space is usually evident between the bridging bone and the vertebral rim on lateral views. The intervertebral joints are not involved and disc height is usually preserved. Ossifying enthesopathy also affects sites around the pelvis (eg posterior pelvic brim, adductor and gluteal insertions); the elbow (triceps insertion); knee (quadriceps and patellar tendon insertions); and calcaneum (Achilles insertion, plantar fascia origin).

Spinal involvement restricts movement but is usually asymptomatic; large anterior ossifications may rarely cause dysphagia. Peripheral lesions are more commonly symptomatic, as in this patient. His radiograph (Figure *b*) shows gross flowing new bone over the posterior calcaneum, "spurring" of the Achilles insertion and plantar fascia origin, and ossification within the plantar fascia. His thoracic radiograph (Figure *a*) confirms extensive involvement as the cause of his limited spinal movement.

The differential diagnosis is seronegative spondarthritis. Syndesmophytes in classic ankylosing spondylitis are usually fine, symmetrical and marginal, originating from the vertebral body rim and closely following the line of the annulus fibres. Spondylitis in psoriasis and chronic Reiter's more commonly results in coarse, non-marginal, asymmetrical syndesmophytes, but these still originate close to the vertebral rim. Both forms of spondylitis associate with sacroiliitis (absent in DISH) and the peripheral enthesopathy often shows proliferative erosive change in early lesions (erosions are not a feature of DISH).

Ossifying enthesopathy resembling DISH can occur as a side effect from retinoic acid derivatives used for skin disorders; presentation is usually with painful peripheral enthesopathy. The associations with obesity and diabetes are unexplained but could relate to increased retinoid and insulin-like growth factors which may stimulate ligamentous and entheseal new bone formation. This patient responded to injection of his plantar fascia insertion site, adoption of shock-absorbing thick-soled shoes (trainers), and weight reduction.

58 Lateral epicondylitis ("tennis elbow").

The origins of extensores carpi radialis brevis and longus ("fist clenchers") at the lateral epicondyle (with brachioradialis origin just above) are the usual site of pain in this common enthesopathy. Both muscles are weak elbow flexors but principally extend the wrist, optimising the action of flexors in power grip. Repetitive gripping in tasks such as housework, machining or using a screwdriver is the usual cause, affecting mainly the dominant arm of middle-aged men and women (rare under 30). The common flexor tendon insertion is similarly the site of pain in less common medial epicondylitis ("golfer's elbow"). Localised tenderness is usually maximal at the epicondyle and pain is reproduced by power grip and resisted wrist extension, as in Figure *b*. Conversely medial epicondylitis pain is reproduced by resisted active wrist flexion and gripping as in Figure *a*. The elbow joint and range of movement is normal.

Pain on resisted active elbow flexion alone suggests a tear of brachialis with less well localized pain and tenderness behind the biceps tendon. This rare lesion may produce a warm, firm mass that is prone to myositis ossificans. Compression of the posterior interosseous nerve (radial tunnel syndrome) may rarely produce lateral elbow and forearm pain; this causes weakness of forearm extensors but no sensory loss.

Management involves avoidance of the provoking activity for at least two months (difficult if occupation-related). Strapping of proximal forearm muscle, epicondylar clasps, cock-up wrist splints and physiotherapy may be helpful, particularly if used early. Local steroid injection commonly improves pain after initial exacerbation (fluorinated steroids are avoided because of skin atrophy). Surgery may be tried for resistant cases.

59 (a) Marked cartilage and bone attrition in whole carpus, radioulnar and distal radioulnar joints; bony ankylosis at radiocarpal, midcarpal and possibly carpometacarpal joints (the trabecular pattern crossing joint lines); large subchondral cyst/geode) in distal radius; loss of joint space at PIPJs; soft tissue swelling at several IPJs; an incidental enchondroma in 3rd metacarpal head.
(b) RA.
(c) Psoriatic arthropathy; ankylosing spondylitis; chronic Reiter's Syndrome; juvenile chronic arthritis (JCA); healed sepsis (including TB); adult-onset Stills (mainly carpometacarpal joints).

Although RA is relatively common it rarely produces bony ankylosis except at the carpus, tarsal joints and cervical spine (unless complicated by sepsis). Ankylosis is more common in seronegative spondarthropathy but is commonly accompanied by bony proliferation. Even in severely damaged RA joints osteophytosis is usually absent or modest ("secondary" OA); exceptions are joints with antecedent primary OA.

Radiographic cysts are common in RA and thought to result from synovial fluid being forced under high pressure through the weakened subchondral plate. They are usually symmetrically distributed, predominating on the proximal side of joints, especially PIPJs, MCPJs, wrists, and big toe MTP and IPJ. They contain fluid, inflamed synovium or both; intraosseous nodules occasionally develop. "Typus robustus" RA patients present a modified radiographic appearance with prominent multiple subarticular cysts, retention of bone density, paucity of erosion and bone attrition, and marginal osteophytosis. Such patients, usually physically active men with prominent nodules, complain of little pain or dysfunction (particularly high intra-articular pressures from zealous physical activity may explain these changes).

Enchondromata are benign tumours of bone (mainly phalanx, humerus) occurring in central locations and destroying cancellous bone. They rarely undergo malignant transformation, particularly when sited in long bones or pelvis.

60 (a) Marfan's Syndrome
(b) Heriditary abnormality of fibrillin.

Marfan's syndrome presents variable phenotypic abnormalities principally in locomotor, ocular, and cardiovascular systems. Inheritance is autosomal dominant; new mutations are uncommon and a family history is usually obtained. The recently described defect is with fibrillin (a glycoprotein of elastic fibres and microfibrils).

Musculoskeletal features include:
- excessive height, with span (outstretched arms) greater than height, and pubis-heel greater than pubis-vertex length, ie low upper/lower segment ratio (normally 0.92).
- arachnodactyly or "spider fingers" (also a feature of homocystinuria and other hereditary disorders), giving an increased radiographic metacarpal index (ratio of length/width of third metacarpal, normally <8.5)
- narrow palm, long thumb and longitudinal laxity of hand, permitting the Steinberg thumb sign (the thumb opposed across the palm within a clenched fist protrudes beyond the ulnar border) and the wrist sign (the thumb and little finger appreciably overlap when wrapped around opposite wrist).
- kyphoscoliosis, chest deformity (especially pigeon-chest), winged scapulae, flat feet.
- hypermobility syndrome due to ligament/tendon laxity, predisposing to arthralgia, recurrent knee effusions, recurrent subluxation/dislocation (especially patellae, hip, mandible)
- typical elongated, asymmetric facial appearance; high-arched palate; asymmetric maldevelopment of lower jaw (Achard's Syndrome).

Ocular involvement is classically ectopia lentis which may advance to subluxation (causing the red, inflamed eye in this patient) or complete dislocation; visible tremor of the iris (iridodonesis) may be evident. High myopia is common, predisposing to retinal detachment, and the sclerae may be blue. The extent of **cardiovascular involvement** is the principal determinant of life expectancy. Cardiovascular problems include:
- congenital atrial septal defect (commonest), coarctation of aorta, patent ductus arteriosus.
- acquired aortic and mitral regurgitation, aortic dissection, pulmonary artery dilatation.

Occasionally peripheral cystic change in the lungs may lead to pneumo-thorax.

The classical syndrome is easy to recognise but difficulty may occur with the more common "forme fruste". Treatment is largely symptomatic; genetic counselling is required.

61 (a) Subchondral lucency with surrounding sclerosis adjacent to weight-bearing surface of medial femoral condyle.
(b) Osteonecrosis (idiopathic osteonecrosis of medial femoral condyle).

Idiopathic medial femoral necrosis occurs in middle-aged or elderly adults, particularly women over age 60. The cause is unknown and unilateral involvement is usual. Onset is spontaneous and acute with unremitting medial knee pain, characteristically worse at night and exacerbated by walking. In the initial stages stiffness, swelling and mild effusion are common; there may be tenderness over the medial condyle and pain on forced knee flexion. Pathologically an island of subchondral bone (1–2cm diameter) separates from the femoral condyle; in 85% this occurs on the medial or central portion of the medial condyle, 15% occur laterally. Symptoms may precede x-ray changes by several months; bone scans are more sensitive and show increased uptake in early cases. The first x-ray change is flattening of the weight-bearing aspect of the medial condyle; eventually a subchondral lucency develops and becomes surrounded by a sclerotic halo of new bone. The osteo-cartilaginous sequestrum may extrude into the joint cavity. MRI can demonstrate the subchondral fracture but may not show cartilage disruption; arthroscopy better demonstrates whether the fragment is in situ, partially detached or free.

Usually symptoms gradually subside and resolve over several months (particularly younger patients who successfully avoid excessive weight-bearing), the lesion healing by bone and fibrocartilaginous repair. However, in c.75% of cases symptomatic medial compartment OA subsequently develops, with or without an intervening period of symptom remission. Treatment in early cases consists of non weight-bearing to encourage healing; the smaller the lesion the greater the chance of resolution. Treatment is conservative if the fragment remains in situ; loose fragments require surgical intervention (removal or fixation).

Osteochondritis dissecans of children/adolescents shows similarities but also differences. Although the knee is most commonly affected other joints may also be involved (hip, ankle, elbow, metatarsal heads, shoulder). Males are more commonly affected (cf. females in the older group) and the condition may be bilateral. Symptoms onset is usually insidious with vague, intermittent, poorly localised aching; persistent rest pain and stiffness aggravated by use then develops. The lateral (cf medial) femoral condyle is usually affected. Locking may result from detachment as a loose body; persistent locking suggests a frequently associated torn meniscus. OA may subsequently develop many years later. Although the condition is also idiopathic, one theory, which accounts for its lateral site, suggests it results from traumatic impact of the tibial spine during violent internal rotation (affected patients reportedly have prominent tibial spines).

Knee osteonecrosis in adults may also be caused by Caisson's disease, alcohol abuse, systemic steroids, sickle-cell anaemia, Gauchers disease and

SLE. However, in these conditions the lesions are generally far removed from the articular surface with more extensive involvement of the lower femur.

62 (a) Figure *a*: digital infarction with gangrene of most finger tips. Figure *b* and *c*: incomplete eye closure; circumoral furrowing; small aperture mouth; pinching of skin around nose.
(b) Scleroderma with severe Raynaud's and digital infarction.

Late-onset Raynaud's with tightness of skin around hands and face is highly suggestive of scleroderma. Her digital gangrene resulted from secondary Raynaud's (this is not a complication of primary Raynaud's). Vasculitis is rare in scleroderma and complement consumption is not usually a feature; in this woman patent blood vessels were confirmed and there was no investigational evidence of vasculitis. Non-specific ANF and rheumatoid factor positivity is common in scleroderma; anti-centromere and anti-SCl_{70} antibodies are more specific. Anticentromere antibody occurs in 50–90% of patients with CREST syndrome and only 10% with systemic sclerosis, its presence therefore conferring a favourable prognosis. Anti SCl_{70} occurs in 20–40% of patients with generalised scleroderma.
    Raynaud's may be classified mechanistically, for example:
• Vasospastic:
    primary Raynaud's disease
    drug-induced (ergot, methysergide)
    phaeochromocytoma
    carcinoid syndrome
• Structural:
    (a) large and medium-sized arteries
    thoracic outlet syndrome
    Takayasu's disease
    atherosclerosis
    (b) small arteries/arterioles
    connective tissue disease (scleroderma, SLE, polymyositis)
    vibration-induced injury
    cold-induced injury
    chemicals (polyvinyl-chloride, bleomycin, vincristine)
• Viscosity problems:
    cryoglobulinaemia, cold agglutinin disease
    cryofibrinogenaemia
    paraproteinaemia, hyperviscosity syndromes
    polycythemia
Small digital arteries of patients with scleroderma show marked intimal hyperplasia (mainly collagen) and often adventitial fibrosis, severely narrowing the lumen. Normal vasoconstrictor response to cold and emotional stimuli superimpose on this anatomic obstruction and may result in complete or near complete occlusion.
    Management of Raynaud's is mainly supportive and hinges on patient education. Avoidance of cold exposure is paramount. Warm clothing (including underwear and hats to maintain central temperature) should obviously be worn outdoors, especially in cold months. Mittens are often warmer than gloves (unless electrically heated). Smoking should be avoided,

as should cold water washing. Any drug therapy is an adjunct to these measures. Calcium channel blockers (nifedipine, diltiazem, verapamil) probably act as anti-vasoconstrictors rather than vasodilators and also reduce platelet activation; ketanserin and dazoxiben (serotonin antagonists) are also effective. Sympathectomy provides only temporary benefit in some patients and is not without risk. Low-dose aspirin (but not dipyridamole) may be beneficial as an antiplatelet agent.

For major crises (pregangrenous or persistant pain) prostacyclin infusion is the treatment of choice; it is a potent vasodilator, promoting healing of digital ulceration and improvement of skin signs. Its effect often lasts for six or more weeks.

63 (a) "Punched-out" marginal and non-marginal erosion; proliferative new bone and "overhanging hook" of Martel.
(b) Gout.
(c) Synovial fluid analysis for urate crystals; serum uric acid; urinary uric acid/creatinine ratio; serum urea and creatinine; fasting lipoproteins; full blood count.

Although there are no specific radiographic changes of gout, occurrence of well-defined "punched-out" erosions away from the joint line with associated bony reaction and "overhanging hook" of Martel sign (and no osteopenia) are characteristic. Such changes take many years to develop and are usually absent at presentation with acute attacks.

The majority (>90%) of patients with primary gout have hyperuricaemia and undersecretion of uric acid due to an inherited isolated renal tubular defect. A small minority are overproducers of uric acid. Features in this man that suggest that he may be an overproducer are:
• early age of onset of gout (in his twenties)
• recurrent renal colic suggesting uric acid stones (more common in overproducers)
• absence of obesity and excess alcohol/beer as common associated risk factors in "young" (<50) men
• no suggestion of drug-induced hyperuricaemia (a risk factor more common in the elderly); no occupational risk of lead poisoning.

Overproducers have very high serum uric acid levels and a high urinary uric acid/creatinine ratio (>0.7). The underlying inherited metabolic defect is variable, but recognised rare enzyme abnormalities include hypoxanthine-guanine phosphoribosyl transferase (HGPRT) deficiency (complete – Lesch-Nyhan syndrome with neurological features; partial – gout and uric acid calculi but little/no neurological impairment); increased activity of phosphoribosyl pyrophosphate synthetase; and glucose-6-phosphatase deficiency. In most overproducers there is increased nucleic acid turnover with a compensatory increase in rate of purine biosynthesis *de novo*; though conditions such as polycythaemia rubra vera, secondary polycythaemia and chronic haemolytic anaemia should be considered in most cases, the underlying cause is unclear.

In this patient gout was confirmed by demonstration of monosodium urate crystals in synovial fluid from an intercritical first MTPJ. He had very high serum uric acid and urinary uric acid/creatinine ratio, and overproduction was confirmed by estimating total 72-hour urinary excretion on a controlled diet. No specific enzyme abnormality was found on erythrocyte studies undertaken at a specialist laboratory. His other investigations were normal, showing no evidence of underlying haematological disease, renal impairment or associated hyperlipidaemia. He was treated successfully with allopurinol but required high doses (900mg) to maintain his serum uric acid in the lower half of the normal range. He was advised to maintain high fluid intake (two to three litres/day) to prevent uric acid nephrolithiasis. He had persistent highly acid urine (common in gout patients) and was therefore also prescribed alkalinising agents (acidity reduces uric acid solubility). His two sons (aged 23 and 21) were investigated for hyperuricaemia; the eldest was found to be an overproducer and was counselled with respect to lifelong prophylaxis with allopurinol.

64 Broadened forefoot; crowding of toes with a deep cleft in the skin between the metatarsal heads; extreme hallux valgus/subluxation with overriding toes; MTPJ subluxation; adventitious bursitis and callosities under metatarsal heads.

The metatarsal region may suffer badly in late RA. Inflammatory weakening, erosion and damage to MTPJ capsules and ligaments lowers resilience against deforming pressure of weight-bearing and shoes and the altered lines of pull of hallux valgus and quintus varus, resulting in characteristic deformity. The proximal phalanges sublux (and eventually dislocate) upwards. This results in (a) clawing and reduced weight-bearing of toes, and (b) forward and upward displacement of the shock-absorbing fibrofatty cushions beneath the metatarsal heads. The latter become relatively unprotected on weight-bearing (pressures increasing by up to 20 × normal) so adventitious bursae and reactive callosities form beneath the metatarsal heads and under the unprotected toe-tips if they take pressure on walking. The first callosity to form is usually under the second metatarsal head ("centre-forward" callosity), usually followed by callosities under the third and fourth lateral metatarsal heads. Dorsal callosities also develop on the clawed toes because of constant rubbing from shoes. Such adventitious bursae and callosities may ulcerate and become secondarily infected; altered, deepened skin clefts secondary to subluxation add to infective problems and chronic sinus formation (sometimes communicating with the MTPJ) may be problematic.

Packing of the toes causes firstly quintus varus, then hallux valgus, leading to over- or underriding of the fifth toe with respect to the fourth. If the toe is very protuberant, shoe fitting may be impossible and amputation may sometimes be undertaken. Corns and bunions are very common and pressure points may also occur along the lateral foot. Relief of abnormal pressure on the central three metatarsal heads often relieves pain and effects disappearance of callus. Non-surgical methods include a felt or rubber pad in the shoe proximal to the central metatarsal heads; a transverse thick leather bar behind the metatarsal heads; inverting the heel or forefoot by medial and lateral shoe wedges respectively; adhesive strapping (shifting the weight more medially on the first metatarsal head); removing callus by nightly hot soaks followed by application of salicylic acid solution; weight reduction; and toe flexor exercises to strengthen intrinsic muscles. Surgery may be necessary for intractable pressure pain beneath the metatarsal heads. Resection of a single metatarsal head is to be avoided since rapid development of similar painful changes in other metatarsals usually follows. The Fowler procedure is often preferred, resecting all metatarsal heads and proximal phalanx bases to pull the toes into a more anatomical position and to resite the displaced fat pads beneath the refashioned metatarsal shafts.

65 Osteoarthritis of index DIPJ (loss of joint space, osteophyte); Paget's disease (expansion/deformity of bone, coarse trabecular pattern, sclerosis) of ring finger proximal phalanx, 5th metacarpal and right femur; Pagetic arthropathy (predominant cartilage loss) ring finger MCPJ and hip.

Paget's disease of bone is of unknown aetiology, occurring in 3% of subjects over age 40 and 10% over age 80. Bone pain and deformity are the principal complaints. Symptoms often relate to a single region but multiple foci (many asymptomatic) is usual. It may affect any bone but frequently affected sites are lumbosacral spine, skull, pelvis, femur and tibia. The clinical and radiographic course is variable and unpredictable.

Paget's disease involves increased osteoclastic bone resorption with compensatory but abnormal increase in osteoblastic activity. New bone is disorganised, lacks normal trabecular pattern, is often increased in size and mechanically weak, predisposing to bowing deformity and fracture. Pain may result from accompanying hypervascularity and intraosseous hypertension (night pain), microfracture or stress fracture. Involvement of subchondral bone may cause "secondary OA" (usually hip, knee) from altered joint architecture and mechanical forces. Mechanical compression from bone enlargement may cause spinal cord and root compression, optic atrophy and deafness; kyphosis, enlarged skull, and bowing of limbs may be readily visible. The cause of pain may be difficult to determine and meticulous history and examination are required. High output cardiac failure and osteogenic sarcoma are rare complications.

Established radiographic findings are characteristic but early lesions may be difficult to interpret. A mixed lytic/sclerotic picture is typical. Marked osteolysis without accompanying sclerosis occurs in "osteoporosis circumscripta" of skull or the V-shaped advancing front of long bones. More usually radiographs show enlargement, cortical thickening, intracortical resorption, loss of cortico-medullary junction and accentuated trabecular markings. Bone scans are sensitive for detecting involved areas. Increased serum alkaline phosphatase is the only abnormal routine biochemical finding (increases also occur in other markers of bone turnover, eg urinary hydroxyproline, pyridinoline collagen cross-links). Symptomatic treatment alone (analgesics, NSAIDs, mechanical measures) is often sufficient, but early aggressive treatment is increasingly being advocated with normalisation of serum alkaline phosphatase the stated goal. Bisphosphonates (etidronate, pamidronate, clodronate), calcitonins and mithramycin are the principal agents that inhibit Paget's disease. The main limiting factor with etidronate and other bisphosphonates is risk of demineralisation, though intermittent high-dose regimes may reduce this problem.

66 (a) Disorganisation with marked carpal attrition; bony debris; soft tissue swelling.
(b) Charcot joint (probably due to syringomyelia).

This man's radiograph shows classic features of a neuropathic (Charcot) joint. Acute onset with pain followed by relatively pain-free chronic swelling and functional disturbance is the typical history. Neurological signs are often subtle and should be carefully sought. Additional peripheral nerve entrapment (median and/or ulnar) secondary to disorganisation and soft tissue swelling at the wrist should be considered and investigated by nerve conduction. If present, intra-articular Yttrium-90 ("medical synovectomy") or surgical decompression may be considered; both, however, are problematic with such deranged anatomy.

Syringomyelia is the usual cause of a neuropathic wrist, elbow or shoulder. Congenital structural deformity of the cervical spine (eg Klippel-Feil deformity) is a rare predisposing factor to syringomyelia (not present in this man). Causes of a Charcot joint at other sites include diabetes, tabo-paresis, congenital insensitivity to pain, leprosy and yaws.

67 (a) The arthrogram shows rupture of a popliteal cyst with "feathering" of contrast into the calf; there is normal filling of the suprapatellar expansion but generalised cartilage loss.
(b) Stop the heparin. Aspirate and inject the knee with steroid. Observe closely for sensory alteration or reduced peripheral pulses (suggesting compartment compression); surgical release if present.

Posterior expansion of the synovium/capsule (popliteal or Baker's cyst) may complicate any condition causing a knee effusion and occasionally occurs as an isolated finding in apparently normal knees. External pressure from tight posterior structures produces a valve mechanism facilitating entry, but not exit, of fluid into the "cyst" during mid flexion; this results in hypertension and further expansion downwards as a calf cyst. Partial resorption of fluid in this "sump" increases its viscosity and inhibits clearance. Additional increase in pressure, as in walking downstairs, may then result in rupture with tracking of irritant fluid into the calf. Rarely chronic expansion and acute rupture occurs upwards into the thigh (posteriorly or anteriorly). A similar phenomenon occurs at other joints, eg wrist, shoulder, hip (also described by Baker).

At the knee acute pain is accompanied by all the signs of a calf deep vein thrombosis (DVT), ie swelling, oedema, warmth, tenderness and positive Homan's sign. The only sign that differentiates a rupture from DVT is bruising around the malleoli following a rupture; this is rare and usually appears after a few days. At presentation a knee effusion may not be evident (rupture decompresses the joint), knee symptoms and signs may be minimal and misdiagnosis as DVT is common. Anticoagulation may cause bleeding into the inflamed calf with subsequent nerve and vessel compression from hypertension within the constraining fascia; permanent muscle damage and gangrene may rarely result.

Confirmation of a ruptured cyst is by arthrography, though if performed late the rupture may have closed. Venography and other investigations for DVT may also be problematic and a negative or equivocal result (as in this case) may not exclude the diagnosis. Furthermore, ruptured cyst and DVT may coexist (the former possibly predisposing to the latter). However, since there are doubts that anticoagulation is mandatory for calf DVT it is prudent to anticoagulate only if investigations are positive.

Standard treatment of a ruptured cyst includes:
• analgesia (simple analgesics, NSAIDs)
• aspiration of the knee to dryness, and injection of long-acting steroid (to temporarily reduce fluid production)
• temporary rest with avoidance of weight bearing (to minimise extreme pressure rises within the joint)

Most seal off fairly quickly following self-decompression. Recurrence is uncommon, perhaps due to scarring and thickening around the rupture site.

This patient improved following cessation of heparin, and aspiration and injection of her knee. Luckily she developed no signs of calf compression and did not require fasciotomy.

68 (a) The patient's right ear is reddened, swollen and flopped forward.
(b) Increased resistance during expiration secondary to collapse of bronchi/bronchioles.
(c) Relapsing polychondritis.

This rare inflammatory chondropathy, presumed to be an autoimmune disease against type II collagen, affects both sexes equally with usual onset in middle-age. Presentation is with inflammation of one or several cartilage sites, sometimes with fever. The course is very variable, ranging from intermittent acute self-limiting episodes ("relapsing polychondritis") to more chronic and insidious disease. Death may result from tracheobronchial or aortic valve dysfunction. Classic target sites and problems include:
• ear cartilage; pain, swelling, erythema, tenderness of upper two-thirds of pinna; weakening later results in floppy, drooping ears (Figure *a*); impaired hearing (swelling of meatus).
• nasal cartilage, with occasional later collapse of distal nose
• joints; arthralgia or mild synovitis, mainly large joints
• larynx; hoarseness, cough, tenderness; rarely marked oedema necessitating tracheostomy
• trachea/bronchial tree; weakness of cartilaginous rings may cause airway collapse during expiration, asphyxsia and infection
• sclera; episcleritis/scleritis
• aortic valve/ring; acute or chronic aortic insufficiency
• costochondral cartilage; pain, tenderness; rarely flail chest

An acute phase response (elevated ESR, viscosity) is usual. Histology of affected structures confirms inflammatory chondropathy (mononuclear-predominant infiltrates, reduced proteoglycan staining, disruption). Joint radiographs may show isolated, diffuse joint space loss. The flow loop is particularly useful for detecting tracheobronchial weakening/collapse during expiration. It shows pressure gradients and respired volumes simultaneously; no-flow points are where the trace is horizontal, the area of the loop mainly reflecting airway resistance.

Short-term high-dose steroids are often used for acute episodes. Cytotoxics (eg azathioprine, methotrexate), dapsone or cyclosporin may be helpful in chronic, frequently relapsing cases.

69 (a) Chondrocalcinosis (predominantly triangular ligament); radiocarpal narrowing, sclerosis, osteophyte and cysts (particularly scaphoid, radius); scapho-lunate dissociation with indentation of scaphoid on radius.
(b) Carpal tunnel syndrome secondary to pyrophosphate arthropathy.

Peripheral nerve entrapment characteristically produces symptoms that predominate or are confined to the early morning (mainly reflecting redistribution of fluid and awkward positioning during sleep). Median nerve entrapment in the carpal tunnel may give:
• paraesthesia, dysaesthesia, numbness or clumsiness of thumb, index and middle fingers (a sensory branch to the radial palm arises proximal to the carpal tunnel)
• aching in the flexor aspect of the forearm
• weakness and wasting of the lateral 2 lumbricals, opponens pollicis, abductor pollicis and flexor pollicis brevis ("LOAF") – usually a late sign (Figure *a*)
Symptoms may be reproduced by rapid percussion over the wrist distal to the proximal skin crease (Tinel's sign) or by forced passive wrist flexion sustained for 1 minute (Phalen's test). Such tests may be positive in normal subjects and definitive diagnosis requires nerve conduction studies. Many cases of carpal tunnel syndrome appear idiopathic, though recognised local and generalised causes include:
• any wrist synovitis/flexor tenosynovitis
• trauma, Colles fracture
• pregnancy
• hypothyroidism
• acromegaly
• amyloid
Generalised conditions may cause bilateral involvement. Thyroid function should be tested in middle-aged/elderly subjects but blind screening is otherwise unwarranted.

The radiographic features of arthropathy in this patient are those of OA, but the atypical site (radiocarpal joint), prominent cysts and scapholunate dissociation are characteristic of "pyrophosphate arthropathy" – a common subset of osteoarthritis in the elderly. Chondrocalcinosis is further support for calcium pyrophosphate crystal deposition. Carpal tunnel syndrome in this condition is principally caused by soft tissue swelling rather than structural change.

Peripheral entrapment of the ulnar nerve at Guyon's canal (formed by the pisohamate ligament bridging pisiform and hamate) may also result from wrist synovitis. Combined median and ulnar entrapment, causing symptoms in all fingers, may occur but is often misdiagnosed as carpal tunnel syndrome in a poor historian. This patient's symptoms improved following intra-articular injection of steroid into her radiocarpal joint (rather than carpal tunnel) and temporary use of a wrist splint at night. She declined the offer of surgical release.

70 (a) Generalised hypermobility syndrome.
(b) Signs of hereditary connective tissue disease, eg abnormal body habitus, high-arched palate, arachnodactyly, easy bruising, lax skin, wide scars etc.

Joint mobility is mainly limited by capsular/ligamentous laxity and muscle tone. It is age-, gender- and race-dependent, being greater in children, females, Afro-Caribbeans, and Asians. About 10% of the general population fall within the lax end of a normal spectrum of joint mobility. Such hypermobility may be advantageous for ballet dancers and gymnasts, and can be increased by training. However, it can predispose to arthralgia (+/- small effusions), enthesopathy, back pain ("loose back syndrome"), kyphoscoliosis, subluxation (eg "loose" patella), and dislocation (especially of the shoulders). Various screening methods have been suggested, including the Beighton score, which examines the following abilities:
• extend little finger >90° (one point each)
• bring back thumb parallel to/touching forearm (one point each)
• extend elbow >10° (one point each)
• extend knee >10° (one point each)
• touch floor with flat hands, legs straight (one point)
   Maximum score = nine (six plus = hypermobile)
   A very small number of hypermobile subjects will have a defined predisposing disease, including Marfan's syndrome (most common), Ehlers-Danlos syndrome, Down's syndrome, acromegaly, and Wilson's disease. Idiopathic "loose joints" is often familial, mainly causing locomotor symptoms in adolescent and young female adults. Association with genital prolapse, varicose veins, and haemorrhoids supports the suggestion of minor collagen abnormalities in such families. Although predisposition to osteoarthritis has been suggested, data on this lacking. Locomotor symptoms often diminish with age as joint mobility declines. Patients should be reassured and advised on posture, joint protection, and exercise to maintain muscle tone.

71 (a) Small blood vessels show dense polymorphonuclear (PMN) cell infiltrates, narrowing, occlusion and vessel wall destruction. Fragmented degenerate PMN nuclei ("nuclear dust") is evident in perivascular areas ("cytoclasis").
(b) Leucocytoclastic vasculitis.

Leucocytoclastic allergic vasculitis (hypersensitivity vasculitis) includes diverse conditions in which vasculitis predominates in smaller vessels, especially post-capillary venules. The skin is the commonest organ targeted, usually without systemic involvement. Cutaneous lesions are often purpuric (usually palpable), though papules, nodules, vesicles, ulcers or urticaria are not uncommon. Lower extremities, buttocks, forearms and hands are common sites. It is usually benign and self-limiting, though occasionally recurrent or chronic.
   A number of aetiological associations have been implicated, including:
• drugs (eg penicillin, sulphonamides, allopurinol, animal serum, vaccines)
• infections (eg Group A Strep., Staph. aureus, Neisseria, Hepatitis B
• connective tissue disease; RA, Sjögren's, SLE, scleroderma, polyarteritis
• malignancy; carcinoma, lymphoma, Waldenström's macroglobulinaemia

• miscellaneous; chronic active hepatitis, ulcerative colitis, primary biliary cirrhosis, bacterial endocarditis, intestinal bypass syndrome
Henoch Schönlein Purpura, Mixed Essential Cryoglobulinaemia and hypocomplementaemic vasculitis are syndromes with systemic involvement in which leukocytoclastic vasculitis is prominent.
This patient improved rapidly following a short course of oral steroids. No cause or trigger to his vasculitis was found.

72 (a) Schmorl's nodes; loss of disc height between L2/L3 with early osteophyte formation.
(b) Scheuermann's disease.

Scheuermann's disease is osteonecrosis of the ring epiphysis of the thoracic vertebrae presenting around puberty, especially in boys. Symptoms are typically vague lower thoracic pain radiating to both loins and relieved by lying flat; a history of preceding strenuous physical/sporting activity is common. Radiographs are initially normal. Over subsequent months pain diminishes but the lower thoracic spine gradually develops rigid kyphotic deformity with rounded shoulders and a flat chest; lower thoracic rigidity is emphasised by increased anterior flexion of higher segments on bending forward. The lateral radiograph now displays irregularity and deficient ossification of vertebral ring epiphyses, especially anteriorly; upper and lower end plates become blurred and irregular with small cup-like indentations (herniating disc material) extending into the spongiosa, appearing more obvious as reactive sclerosis develops. These Schmorl's nodes are accompanied by variable intevertebral space narrowing and anterior wedging. The ring then completes its ossification, extending as a dense horizontal line parallel with the vertebral body; as growth finishes the ring fuses with the body and the deformity is permanent. Compensatory increased cervical and lumbar lordosis may produce excessive strain and subsequent degenerative changes later in adult life, mainly at the lumbosacral junction.
Strict bed rest is advised during the early painful phase. A plaster cast is occasionally used to reduce deformity. As pain settles hyperextension exercises are important. A brace and/or surgery may be considered in severe cases.

73 (a) Pustular psoriasis or keratoderma blenorrhagica.
(b) Proliferative erosive enthesopathy (with accompanying new bone) at the plantar fascia origin.
(c) Reiter's disease.

Acute-onset asymmetric oligoarthritis of lower limb joints, with calcaneal enthesopathy ("lover's heel"), in a young man is the classic picture of acute Reiter's disease. Enquiry should include urogenital or gastrointestinal disturbance. Urethritis occurs as part of the reactive syndrome and may follow (but not precede) dysentery-triggered Reiter's. This patient admitted to an episode of non-specific urethritis two weeks before (following unprotected intercourse in a foreign port). He had no urethritis or conjunctivitis at presentation.
Relatively painless/asymptomatic mucosal lesions (mouth, urethra, cervix) are often present if sought in Reiter's. Keratoderma is uncommon

but usually striking. It presents as a painless papulo-squamous eruption on soles and palms (rarely trunk, scalp or elsewhere) and is clinically and histologically indistinguishable from pustular psoriasis (chronic Reiter's and psoriasis additionally share nail dystrophy and radiographic characteristics of sacroiliitis/spondylitis). Acute and chronic enthesopathy (inflammation at sites of ligament/tendon/capsule insertion into bone) is a characteristic feature of spondyloarthropathies. Common symptomatic sites include Achilles tendon and plantar fascia insertions; enthesopathy of symphysis pubis, ischium, and iliac crest is usually asymptomatic (but often apparent radiographically in chronic Reiter's). Enthesopathy (and arthropathy) in spondyloarthropathies is erosive but accompanied by new bone formation (florid in some chronic lesions); such "proliferative" erosions usually permit distinction from other causes of enthesopathy (eg RA, repetitive trauma). Diffuse idiopathic skeletal hyperostosis may produce similar impressive ossifying enthesopathy but without erosion.

The classic triad of arthritis, urethritis, and conjunctivitis occurs in about a third of patients with Reiter's. The remaining "forme frustes" (reactive arthritis) are identified on the basis of typical oligoarthritis accompanied by one or more of the following:
- diarrhoea
- urethritis, cervicitis, mouth ulcers
- ocular inflammation
- enthesitis
- keratoderma blennorrhagica

The commonest triggering microbial agents are Salmonella, Shigella, Yersinia, Campylobacter and Chlamydia. The typical arthritis follows within two to three weeks as an acute, asymmetric, additive oligoarthritis targeting lower limb joints (first MTPJ, ankles, knees, toes); involvement of upper limb joints and spine is unusual (never in isolation). Synovitis may be florid. "Sausage digits" result from combined synovitis, enthesopathy, tenosunovitis and periostitis in a whole ray. The acute attack inevitably settles over several months but over half subsequently develop chronic Reiter's syndrome with radiographic sacroiliitis. Differential diagnosis of acute Reiter's may include septic arthritis (especially gonococcal), crystal arthropathies, sarcoidosis, erythema nodosum and RA. Usual differentiation, however, is from other spondylarthropathies (especially psoriasis) and reactive arthropathies (rheumatic fever, AIDS-associated reactive arthritis).

NSAIDs and patient education are sufficient treatment in most cases. Sulphasalazine, methotrexate and azathioprine may be indicated for severe, persistent arthropathy. Treatment of triggering infection (particularly chlamydia – tetracycline) may be required. Prolonged antibiotic therapy in those with postdysenteric or idiopathic Reiter's is unlikely to be useful.

74 (a) Joint space narrowing with prominent cysts variably affecting radio-carpal, midcarpal, scaphotrapezoid, first CMCJ, and all MCPJs.
(b) Liver stained with Perl's Prussian blue showing distortion of architecture and increased iron deposition.
(c) Haemochromatosis with arthropathy.

Arthropathy develops in c.50% of patients with haemochromatosis. Arthralgia is a common early symptom that may predate the diagnosis and occurrence of classic features (bronze pigmentation, hepatomegaly, diabetes, heart failure) by many years. Chronic arthralgia is the dominant symptom, particularly affecting MCPJs, wrists, shoulders, hips, knees and ankles. Chronic synovitis is unusual though acute attacks (due to associated calcium pyrophosphate crystal deposition) occur in up to 30%.

Radiographic changes resemble OA except for:
• distribution: predominant MCPJ, wrist, shoulder and ankle involvement is rare in OA
• relative paucity of osteophyte
• sometimes rapid bone attrition and fragmentation at hip (resembling extensive avascular necrosis)
• concurrence of chondrocalcinosis (c.60%)

The radiographic features and young age for development of OA or chondrocalcinosis usually suggest the diagnosis. Serum ferritin levels are grossly raised and liver function tests are usually deranged. The diagnosis is confirmed by liver biopsy (Figure b).

This man was treated by regular venesection to reduce his initially very high serum ferritin to subnormal levels. Screening of his family revealed a presymptomatic sister who was also treated by venesection. As is usual, his joint symptoms persisted despite treatment of his haemochromatosis.

75 (a) Right-sided pleural effusion.
(b) Rice bodies; joint fluid aspirates (initially described in tuberculous effusions, but now mainly seen with RA).
(c) Fibrin and cells.

Rice bodies, so-called because of similarity to polished rice grains, are usually only aspirated if large gauge needles are used (eg during arthroscopy). They show no correlation with chronicity or severity of RA. Some consider them potential inflammatory agents and recommend removal by lavage or treatment by intra-articular steroid.

Pleural effusions complicating RA predominate in middle-aged men and may be unilateral or bilateral. Most are asymptomatic and resolve spontaneously; large/bilateral effusions may cause breathlessness. Other causes of effusion need exclusion and aspiration (for culture, cytology, biochemical analysis) is usually required. Characteristics of RA effusions include:
• low glucose (10–50 mg/dl)
• raised protein (>4 g per dl)
• increased cells, occasional giant "comet" cells (rhagocytes)
• greatly elevated lactic dehydrogenase
• depressed CH_{50}

Low sugar, probably reflecting impaired glucose transport into the pleural space, also occurs with sepsis (particularly TB) which may coexist. Systemic treatment of RA (ie second-line drug therapy) usually results in reduction/resolution of the effusion.

76 Neuropathic (Charcot) joint.

The radiograph shows typical changes of a Charcot joint – florid cartilage and bone attrition, fragmentation and disruption of normal architecture (joint "disorganisation"). Other classic features include fractures, massive soft tissue swelling, effusion and ossific debris. The bone response is variable, ranging from florid proliferative new bone ("hypertrophic") to complete absence of a reparative response ("atrophic" resorptive Charcot joint). Acute onset with swelling and pain is typical, though pain is often less severe than might be expected and may be absent particularly once disorganisation is established. Classic clinical signs include instability with increased range of movement and crepitus. As the bones collapse loss of arches with eventual convexity of the volar surface may produce a "rocker" foot.

The mechanism remains unclear. Autonomic dysfunction, resulting in increased blood flow to bone and synovium, may be more important than reduced pain and proprioception (a "hot" bone scan precedes joint abnormality). Clinical signs of underlying neuropathy may be subtle.

Diabetes is the commonest cause, target sites being the mid, fore- and hindfoot (forefoot disease usually atrophic/resorptive; mid and hindfoot disease mainly destructive/hypertrophic). Involvement is usually unilateral and not uncommonly follows overt trauma. Other joints are rarely affected. Radiographically the principal differential diagnosis is sepsis. Loss of cortical outline is usual in sepsis whereas in neuroarthropathy bony margins produced by fragmentation remain well defined.

Management is difficult and often complicated by other complications of diabetic neuropathy (eg ulcers). Careful foot hygiene and appropriate supporting footwear are paramount.

Other causes of neuropathic joints include:
• syringomyelia (shoulder, elbow, wrist, cervical spine)
• tabes dorsalis (knee, ankle, thoracolumbar spine)
• congenital insensitivity to pain (ankle)
• leprosy, yaws (ankle, feet, hands)

77 (a) Corneal arcus (senilis) and tendon xanthomata.
(b) Hyperlipoproteinaemia (Type II, hypercholesterolaemia).
(c) Premature atherosclerosis and ischaemic heart disease.

Type II hyperlipoproteinaemia is a rare inherited disorder characterised by:
• marked hypercholesterolaemia
• corneal arcus
• tendon xanthomata, tendinitis, tenosynovitis
• large joint migratory arthritis
• accelerated atherosclerosis

Presentation is usually with migratory arthritis in childhood (homozygotes) or as a young adult (heterozygotes). The arthritis targets knees and ankles (less commonly hips, elbows, wrists) and is characterized by both synovitis and periarticular inflammation, often with overlying erythema. Children are often febrile and have aortic systolic murmurs and an elevated ESR, leading to common misdiagnosis of rheumatic fever. Attacks last from a few days to a week and recur at irregular intervals often years apart. Cholesterol crystals are not found in synovial fluid and the mechanism of the inflammation is unclear. Achilles tendinitis and tenosynovitis, without systemic upset, are often prominent problems in adult heterozygotes. Despite recurrent inflammation in joints and tendons there are no long-term locomotor sequelae.

Arthritis and tendinitis may predate other clinical manifestations so that xanthomata and corneal arcus are not always present to suggest the diagnosis. Early intervention in children and young adults with (a) diet (low cholesterol and saturated fat, high polyunsaturated fat) and (b) cholestyramine resin is often effective in normalising plasma cholesterol, phospholipids and low density lipoproteins and countering predisposition to atherosclerosis.

78 (a) Narrowing and anterior osteophyte, with minor end plate irregularity and posterior osteophyte, affecting C5/6 and C67 intervertebral joints. (b) Cervical spondylosis with C6 root compression and carpal tunnel syndrome.

Spinal "degenerative" change (intervertebral disc narrowing, vertebral body osteophyte, apophyseal joint osteoarthritis, changes in laminal arches) is an almost universal accompaniment to ageing. It particularly targets lower cervical and lumbar segments and is apparent on x-rays in most adults over age 30. Poor correlation between radiographic change and symptoms results in continuing difficulty over definition of "spondylosis".

Mechanical effects of cervical spondylosis may result in:

(a) **Pain.** This is poorly localised to the neck and shoulders and arises from ligaments, muscles, discs or joints. Pain is often referred to the occiput, nuchal muscles and superior aspect of shoulders. Less common pain patterns include retro-orbital and temporal pain (C2–C3); upper thoracic and interscapular pain; anterior chest pain (C6, C7); and widespread upper limb aching (often mistaken for periarticular lesions such as epicondylitis, rotator cuff tears). The pain is worsened by neck movement (often in one plane) or prolonged lifting, and usually relieved by rest. Neurological signs are absent but hyperalgesia at the referred site (non-dermatomal pattern) is common.

(b) **Cervical radiculopathy.** Nerve root compression due to apophyseal osteophye usually occurs at the C5–C7 level. Sensory symptoms (shooting pain, paraesthesia, hyperaesthesia) follow a segmental pattern and are more common than lower motor neurone weakness. Reflexes may be reduced (biceps and supinator – C5/6 lesions; triceps – C7). Coughing, straining, or sneezing may exacerbate symptoms; sustained shoulder abduction (as in this patient) often temporarily improves a C6 lesion.

(c) **Cervical myelopathy.** The cervical expansion leads to a relatively tight fit for the cord in the lower cervical spine, making it particularly vulnerable to pressure from vertebral osteophyte, retrolisthesis (posterior slide) and disc protrusion.

Osteophytic encroachment on vertebral arteries can further compromise cord function. It usually presents with slowly progressive disability; clumsiness, weakness or dysaesthesia of the hands, and an upper motor neurone gait disturbance.

The distribution of this patient's pain, with exacerbation by neck movements and prolonged carrying, sounded typical of spondylosis. Subsequent development of sensory disturbance over the posterior forearm, thumb and index finger, with reduced biceps and supinator jerks, fit well with a C6 root lesion; the sofa position she described (shoulder abduction) would be expected to relieve the pressure on this root. The early morning timing of her most recent symptoms, however, suggested peripheral nerve entrapment and provocation tests reproduced symptoms consistent with carpal tunnel syndrome. This patient therefore has the "double crush" syndrome – proximal root compression (cervical radiculopathy) makes the distal fibres more susceptible to peripheral entrapment. The combination of cervical spondylosis with carpal tunnel syndrome is most common, though ulnar or radial entrapment may also occur.

Intervertebral changes of spondylosis are evident on lateral radiographs but oblique views are required for foraminal encroachment. Electromyography and nerve conduction studies confirmed "double crush" syndrome in this patient. Local injection abolished her carpal tunnel symptoms and her neck problems improved following physiotherapy (aimed at improving muscle strength and range of movement using passive mobilisation techniques), advice on posture and weight reduction.

79 (a) Scalp infarcts crossing the mid-line (unlike Herpes Zoster); prominent, thickened temporal artery.
(b) Giant-cell (cranial or temporal) arteritis (GCA).
(c) High-dose steroids, possibly plus cytotoxics and low-dose aspirin.

GCA is restricted to patients over 55 years old. It may involve any medium or large artery, but shows predilection for aortic branches to the head and neck. The temporal arteries are superficial and accessible, and are therefore the usual sites where signs are manifested.
Local manifestations depend on the artery involved and include:
• headache – typical (temporal) or posterior (occipital)
• sudden blindness (opthalmic)
• transient diplopia due to extraocular muscle paresis
• jaw pain (claudication) on chewing (facial) – unlike temporomandibular joint pain this is limited to chewing (not talking or opening the mouth wide).
Aortic involvement rarely produces symptoms of an aortic arch syndrome. Clinically evident necrosis resulting from arterial occlusion is rare but may affect the scalp or tongue.

Systemic manifestations include anorexia, weight loss and fever, and symptoms identical to polymyalgia rheumatica. Investigations usually reveal a marked acute-phase response with anaemia (normochromic, normocytic), thrombocytosis, greatly elevated ESR and CRP, and mild abnormalities of liver function. Systemic features may predominate and result in presentation with unexplained anaemia, pyrexia of unknown origin, or a picture simulating occult cancer.

Although serious eye manifestations may develop acutely most patients have preceding local or systemic symptoms for several months. The greatly raised ESR and clinical picture should suggest the diagnosis and result in immediate treatment (this is a rheumatological emergency). Absolute confirmation is by biopsy of a symptomatic or clinically uninvolved temporal artery; however, the arteritis is typically patchy and a negative biopsy does not *exclude* the diagnosis. Positive histology may show fragmentation and infiltration of the internal elastic lamina by histiocytes, lymphocytes and giant cells, with subsequent narrowing and occlusion of the lumen. Biopsies may be positive for up to a week after initiation of treatment.

GCA responds dramatically to prednisolone, but higher doses than those used for polymyalgia rheumatica are needed. A starting dose of 30mg of prednisolone is usual, though higher doses (40–60mg) are used if visual symptoms are present. Low-dose aspirin may reduce the incidence of vascular occlusion. Doses are reduced once the inflammation is effectively suppressed (as evident by symptoms and ESR) and cytoxics (azathioprine, cyclophosphamide, methotrexate) are commonly given as an adjunct and as steroid sparing agents. Treatment is usually continued for between one and two years; GCA is usually a single shot disease and recurrences (unlike in polymyalgia) are rare.

This woman was immediately given prednisolone (60mg daily) with low-dose aspirin. Tragically, however, she developed bilateral blindness within 24 hours of admission.

80 (a) Acute crystal synovitis (gout) is most likely but septic arthritis requires exclusion.
(b) Synovial fluid examination for crystals; Gram stain and culture of synovial fluid, blood and urine; chest x-ray.
(c) Parenteral flucloxacillin (with or without cefotaxime) while awaiting culture results.

Clinically, acute crystal arthritis and sepsis can appear identical (synovitis, erythema, fever, systemic upset), and both may coexist; therefore in acute monoarthritis both need investigation. Both trigger an acute phase response (peripheral leukocytosis; elevated ESR, CRP) and associate with turbid synovial fluid/pus with elevated cell count (>95% polymorphs). Appropriate synovial fluid analysis is therefore required for accurate diagnosis.

In adults sepsis in previously normal joints is unusual without preceding trauma or compromised immunity (eg diabetes, renal failure). More typically sepsis superimposes on pre-existing arthropathy, particularly RA and OA. Acute crystal synovitis, however, commonly occurs in previously asymptomatic joints. The commonest form at the knee is "pseudogout" due to calcium pyrophosphate crystal deposition; this usually affects patients over age 60 and commonly (but not always) associates with radiographic chondrocalcinosis. Gout also affects the knee, sometimes as the presenting joint but more usually one to two decades after initial attacks in the feet. In this man acute gout would be the most likely diagnosis.

Acute attacks of gout may be triggered by:
• trauma
• intercurrent illness/surgery
• acute gout at another site ("cluster attack")
• initiation of drug therapy (eg allopurinol, uricosurics, diuretics)
• blood transfusion/parenteral fluid
• dietary or alcohol excess ("binging")
• starvation diet, dehydration

Triggering of the acute phase response (intercurrent illness, surgery, attacks at other joints) is a common predisposing factor and exacerbation of this man's asthma is probably relevant in causation. However, respiratory infection with bacteraemia and predisposition to sepsis (particularly if on high steroid doses) also requires consideration. In situations where sepsis is a possibility (eg post-operative attacks, compromised immunity, unwell patient) even if crystals have been identified, treatment for sepsis should be instituted pending the culture results 24–48 hours later. Misdiagnosis and delay in treating sepsis even by 48 hours can be catastrophic for the joint and patient. In adults Staphylococcus aureus is the commonest organism (gonococcus requires consideration particularly in younger subjects); in the elderly or compromised streptococci and Gram negative are significantly frequent. When no organisms are seen by Gram stain empirical treatment therefore usually includes flucloxacillin with or without another agent to broaden the spectrum of cover.

This man was admitted. His chest x-ray showed no evidence of occult infection. Monosodium urate crystals were identified in the knee aspirate and no organisms were seen on Gram staining; cultures of synovial fluid, blood and urine were subsequently negative. He was given parenteral flucloxacillin and cefotaxime, daily knee aspiration, and a quick-acting NSAID. His attack settled quickly, antibiotics were stopped after 48 hours and he was rapidly mobilised.

81 (a) Synovitis of the MCPJs and swan-neck deformities.
(b) Boutonniere deformity; subluxation of the MCPJs; Z-thumb deformity; mallet finger; mutilans.

In the figure synovitis of the MCP joints is evident but the most obvious abnormality is swan-neck deformities of the fingers. Other deformities include subluxation of the MCP joints with ulnar deviation, Boutonniere deformity and a Z-thumb deformity. The swan-neck deformity is characterised by hyperextension of the proximal interphalangeal joint and flexion of the distal joint. Its primary basis is thought to be a synovitis of the flexor tendon sheaths resulting in restriction of interphalangeal joint flexion. The interossei become shortened to produce flexion of the MCP which is accompanied by intrinsic muscle shortening tending to pull the PIP into hyperextension. The profundus tendon now bow-strings over the extended PIP contributing to the final part of the deformity, the flexion of the DIPJ is felt to be a secondary phenomenon.

In the Boutonniere deformity the hyperplastic synovium bulges between the central and lateral extensor tendons. The capsular and bony insertions of the central tendon are stretched and the tendon is unable to extend the middle phalanx. The transverse fibres that connect the lateral tendons to the central tendon are weakened by the synovial invasion. This allows the lateral tendons to displace volarward, anterior to the axis of the PIP, becoming flexors of the joint. Furthermore, all their force is exerted on the distal phalanx which becomes hyperextended.

Deformities at the MCPJ are caused by disruption of the extensor tendon expansion which weakens the supporting collateral ligaments. Furthermore, the flexor tendon sheath is disrupted, and the flexor tendon becomes displaced volarward and ulnarward, exerting a further deforming force. As a result, the deformity is characterised by ulnar drift, volar subluxation, and contracted ulnar intrinsics, producing flexion contracture of the MCPJ. This triad of ulnar drift, palmar subluxation and dislocation is the most prevalent deformity of the rheumatoid hand.

The thumb Boutonniere deformity or Z deformity is the most common thumb deformity in RA. The extensor pollicis longus tendon and the abduc tor expansion are displaced ulnarward, and the lateral portion of the expansion, which is a continuation of the flexor brevis and abductor brevis is displaced radial-ward in relation to the MCPJ. The attachment of the extensor brevis to the base of the proximal phalanx is stretched and becomes ineffective. Flexion deformity of the MCPJ ensues. The displaced extensors exert maximal power on the IPJ which becomes hyperextended. With further destruction the MCPJ becomes disorganized and subluxation occurs. In addition, the IPJ becomes unstable for lateral pinch.

Another common deformity is the isolated flexion deformity of the DIP which results in the so-called mallet finger, which is caused by an avulsion/stretching of the extensor tendon.

82 (a) Upward migration/subluxation of the humoral head and loss of glenohumeral joint (GHJ) space with subchondral sclerosis.
(b) Chronic rotator cuff rupture.
(c) The rotator cuff plays a critical role in stabilising the GHJ and is formed by the subscapularis (anterior), supraspinatus, infraspinatus, and teres minor (all posterior).

Chronic rotator cuff rupture causes upward migration of the humeral head, which may then impinge on the undersurface of the acromium (the normally intervening cuff having disrupted). Secondary degenerative changes (sclerosis, pressure erosion, cysts, and osteophytes) commonly develop on the humeral head and undersurface of acromium, and in the remaining functional part of the GHJ ("cuff-tear arthropathy").

The rotator cuff muscles and tendons play a critical role in stabilising the GHJ, acting in co-ordination to fix the head in the glenoid and to cause the head to descend as the humerus abducts (radiographic diminution of subacromial space may be more evident in abduction). In young adults considerable force is required to tear the cuff, eg major direct trauma, unexpected falls on an outstretched arm, or during sporting activities. Possibly due to predisposing degenerative tendinitis and reduced vascularity, less force is required in older subjects, tears often appearing "idiopathically" or following relatively minor trauma or unusual exertion. Tears may be partial or complete (ie involving the full thickness and floor of the overlying subacromial bursa). As with degenerative tendinitis the supraspinatus is most commonly affected. Partial tears usually affect the underside of the tendon near its insertion; non-progressive pain, maximal around the upper arm, develops within a few days and relates to only one or a few movements; any weakness relates to pain inhibition. Acute full-thickness tears often result in immediate pain and muscle spasm, with marked weakness of often several GHJ movements. Infiltration of local anaesthetic abolishes pain but not weakness. Localised wasting may develop (cf global wasting of GHJ arthropathy). Full tears can exist for years with only minor symptoms, especially in elderly subjects with restricted functional demands.

Apart from possible superior migration of the humeral head, radiographs are usually normal in the acute stage. Complete tears may be confirmed by GHJ arthrography showing leakage of contrast into the subacromial bursa; small tears may show as irregularities. MRI imaging readily demonstrates partial or complete tears and is now the investigation of choice.

83 (a) Taut, shiny skin; ill-defined skin creases; areas of hypopigmentation; finger pallor due to Raynaud's.
(b) Scleroderma.

Skin changes in scleroderma inevitably first affect fingers and hands. Initially the skin appears shiny, taut and occasionally erythematous; skin creases (especially IPJ) become less prominent and hair growth is sparse. Skin of the face and neck is usually next involved, resulting in a hypomobile, pinched facies with thin, pursed lips and radial furrowing around the mouth. Skin tightening/thickening may limit mouth opening and impair dental hygiene. Skin changes may remain restricted to fingers, hands and face and be relatively mild. Extension to forearms is followed by spontaneous arrest of progression (limited scleroderma) or by often rapid centripetal spread to upper arms, shoulders, anterior chest, back, abdomen and legs (generalised scleroderma). In late disease mixed hypo- and hyperpigmentation ("salt and pepper" appearance), atrophy of skin and subcutaneous tissues, and fragility and laxity of the superficial dermis may develop.

In generalised scleroderma, the rate of progression of skin changes is variable, ranging from several months to years; episodes of rapid progression often alternate with periods of quiescence. In contrast, limited scleroderma is very slowly but inexorably progressive, with minimal/no change evident from year to year. Development can be summarized into three stages:
1. An early oedematous phase.
2. A phase of dermal thickening and skin tightness.
3. Atrophic phase with contracture.

Tightening and thickening of skin reflects accumulation of excess collagen (types I and III, in the same proportions as normal skin) and extracellular matrix (including glycosoaminoglycans, fibronectin). Early lesions show increased hyalinised collagen in lower dermis and upper subcutaneum with perivascular and interstitial infiltrates of lymphocytes and histiocytes. Later atrophic changes include epidermal thinning with loss of rete pegs and dermal appendages.

Other disorders with proximal skin thickening which may enter the differential diagnosis of systemic sclerosis/scleroderma include the following:
1. Disorders with skin thickening on fingers/hands:
   digital sclerosis of diabetes
   reflex sympathetic dystrophy
   mycosis fungoides
   amyloidosis
   chronic vibration injury
   bleomycin
   polyvinyl chloride disease
2. Disorders with generalised skin thickening but typically sparing fingers/hands:
   scleromyxoedema
   eosinophilic fasciitis
   generalised morphoea
   pentazocine-induced scleroderma
   amyloidosis

3. Disorders characterised by asymmetric skin changes:
   morphoea
   linear scleroderma (*coup de sabre*)
4. Disorders characterised by internal organ involvement similar to systemic sclerosis:
   primary biliary cirrhosis
   collagenous colitis
   infiltrative cardiomyopathy.
   idiopathic pulmonary fibrosis
   primary pulmonary hypertension
5. Disorders characterised by Raynaud's phenomenon (Q. and A. 62)

84 (a) The pupil is irregular and scalloped due to secondary tethering of the iris by synechiae; this is characteristic of iridocyclitis or anterior uveitis.
(b) Juvenile chronic arthritis (JCA).
(c) Antinuclear antibody (ANA).

The classic triad of eye involvement in JCA includes anterior uveitis, band keratopathy and secondary cataract. Eye disease particularly complicates oligoarticular JCA (20%), especially targeting ANA-positive girls. Acute uveitis presents with pain, redness and decreased visual acuity. Chronic uveitis, however, is usually insidious in onset and asymptomatic. Routine opthalmologic examination should therefore be undertaken in every child with pauciarticular JCA (yearly if ANA-negative; three-monthly for the first five years if ANA-positive). Uveitis becomes bilateral within a year in two-thirds of cases. Early signs are increased cells in the anterior chamber or punctate keratitic precipitates on the posterior cornea. Treatment with steroid eye-drops and mydriatics is usually readily effective. However, if missed, posterior synechiae may produce an irregular, poorly reactive pupil and eventually predispose to secondary glaucoma, cataract and permanent visual loss/blindness. Band keratopathy is considered a pathognomic secondary problem and results from calcification of Bowmans Layer, starting at each limbus and working across the cornea to join as a single band; slit-lamp examination is required to detect early signs but it is eventually visible on inspection.

85 (a) Schmorl's nodes; anterior osteophyte/"enthesophyte"; facet joint osteoarthritis (narrowing, sclerosis); calcified (atherosclerotic) aorta.
(b) Degenerative changes in facet joints (facet joint syndrome).

Cartilage covering the vertebral end plates and the nucleus pulposus of the intervertebral disc are subject to age-related degenerative change (intervertebral osteochondrosis). Fissuring may facilitate herniation of nucleus material into adjacent cancellous bone. Bone reaction limits the extruded nucleus pulposus tissue within a fibrous/bony encasement, producing a Schmorl's node. The prolapsed material may change to cartilage or ossify. An important consequence of herniation is disc thinning, posterior displacement of the axis of motion and increased stress on the posterior facets, producing osteoarthritis of posterior facet joints (as in this case). Schmorl's nodes also result from congenitally wide openings/defects in the vertebral end plates; this produces nodes, uniform in size shape and situation (invariably opposite the site of greatest nuclear expansion), at multiple levels in young adults (cf larger, irregular, single or few "degenerative" herniations in older subjects).

Syndesmophytes (in seronegative spondarthritis) are vertically oriented bony excrescences which follow the line of the outer annulus fibres, predominate antero-laterally and eventually bridge the intervertebral space. In contrast osteophyte (in spondylosis deformans) arises several mm from the discovertebral junction, is often triangular in shape and horizontal at least in its initial part. In diffuse idiopathic hyperostosis (DISH) thick, flowing new bone develops in the anterior longitudinal ligament, often with clear separation from the anterior edges of the vertebral bodies. The synovial apophyseal (facet) joints comprise the superior and inferior articular processes of the posterior neural arch. During flexion/extension and rotation of the spine gliding motion occurs at these joints; the encasing capsular/ligamentous structure tightens at the extremes of movement and is particularly vulnerable to tearing injury, with secondary facet joint subluxation, by hyperextension stresses. Predisposing factors to such injury include:
• mechanical stress (obesity; excessive bending/lifting)
• acute lumbosacral angle (> the normal 120°) caused by forward-tilting of pelvis (eg wearing high heels; extra lumbar vertebra; compensatory lumbar lordosis secondary to increased dorsal kyphosis)
• ageing/degenerative change
• loss of intervertebral disc
• vertical disposition of articular facets

In facet joint syndrome the facets sublux, the inferior displacing upward to impinge on the inferior vertebral notch of the above vertebra where it may compress the nerve root, the superior facet impinging on the lower vertebral body and become weight-bearing. As a result the facets and notches become sclerosed and the facet joints develop increasing changes of osteoarthritis (narrowing, sclerosis, irregularity, osteophyte). Initially, ligament/capsule strain and subluxation may manifest with local symptoms, particularly accentuated by hyperextension. Later nerve root compression may cause sciatica and neurological abnormality. Eventually chronic or intermittent symptoms of facet joint osteoarthritis may be superimposed. Facet subluxation may occasionally strain the intervetebral discs sufficiently to cause rupture; most commonly, however, disc protrusion accompanies flexion injury.

86 (a) Ill-defined cortical outlines; marked subperiosteal resorption on distal aspects of proximal phalanx; mild asymetric PIPJ joint space loss; calcification/ossicle adjacent to PIPJ.
(b) Secondary hyperparathyroidism (secondary to renal failure) resulting in phosphate retention and decreased $1:25\text{-}(OH)_2\text{-}D$ production.

Renal osteodystrophy is characterised by a variable combination of osteitis fibrosa cystica, osteomalacia, osteoporosis and osteosclerosis. The typical radiographic appearance of advanced renal osteodystrophy is a patchy mixture of osteopenia and osteosclerosis. Osteomalacia is thought primarily to result from decreased $1:25\text{-}(OH)_2\text{-}D$ production, exacerbated by increased

aluminium deposition in bone (inhibiting osteoblastic activity) from the water and dialysate. Decreased 1:25-$(OH)_2$-D production, reduced renal phosphate clearance and low calcium levels stimulate secondary parathormone secretion which may lead to osteitis fibrosa, characterised clinically by bone pains and predisposition to fracture. Radiographs may reveal:
• generalised osteopenia (common; exacerbated by acidosis, malnutrition)
• subperiosteal resorption (especially middle phalanges, clavicles)
• bone cysts ("brown-tumours")
Osteosclerosis is usually localised and often most obvious in lumbar vertebrae where alternating bands of sclerosis and osteopenia produce the "rugger-jersey" spine.

Joint symptoms in chronic renal dialysis patients may result from crystal synovitis (urate, calcium pyrophosphate, oxalate); calcific periarthritis; sepsis; uraemic osteoarthropathy; and rarely subchondral collapse secondary to metabolic bone disease.

87 (a) Marked osteophytosis (femoral, inferior patella); patellar sclerosis. The interosseous distance ("joint space") appears relatively preserved.
(b) Marked narrowing of the lateral patellofemoral compartment is now apparent, with patellar sclerosis and cyst formation.
(c) Patellofemoral OA.

Pain arising at the knee is generally well localised, the patient readily pointing to the site of maximal discomfort. Intracapsular problems cause anterior knee pain with further localisation according to the compartment involved (patellofemoral – retropatellar; medial tibiofemoral – anteromedial; lateral tibiofemoral – anterolateral).

The patellofemoral compartment is maximally stressed when weight-bearing on the flexed knee. Patellofemoral pain is therefore characteristically worsened and often confined to walking up, and particularly down, stairs and inclines. Another characteristic symptom is progressive aching while sitting with knees flexed (the "movie sign" – the patient being unable to watch a movie through without standing up to relieve pain). Stressing the compartment by the "grind" test (Figure *a*) or by getting the patient to tense the quadriceps (particularly while the examiner pushes the patella down towards the foot) will reproduce the pain.

The patellofemoral and medial tibiofemoral compartments are commonly targeted in OA, both separately and in combination. The lateral compartment is rarely targeted in isolation but commonly becomes involved with severe disease in the other two compartments (ie. tricompartmental OA). Osteophyte is well visualised on the lateral 20 degree flexion radiograph but the interosseous distance is often difficult to assess. The skyline view shows narrowing more clearly; usually, as in this case, the lateral facet and condyle are predominantly affected.

This patient's symptoms were improved by a combined approach involving weight reduction, simple analgesics, patella strapping (pulling the patella medially), regular quadriceps exercises, and use of shoes with thick cushioned soles.

88 (a) Extensor tendon slip or rupture.
(b) Extensor tendon slip.

Inability to actively extend little and ring fingers (with full passive extension) implies an extensor tendon or muscle problem. Although this could reflect tendon rupture (commonly affecting these fingers; usually occurring around the distal radio-ulnar joint) support across the metacarpal heads holds the tendons in their normal dorsal position and corrects the problem (Figure *b*; this would have no effect on tendon rupture). In RA, psoriasis and other inflammatory arthropathies rupture of the ulnar aspect of the MCPJ capsule permits the common extensor tendons to slip to the ulnar side of the metacarpal heads, limiting finger extension and causing ulnar deviation (the tendon itself is not ruptured). Surgical repair of the MCPJ capsule is usually effective.

89 (a) A radiolucent line around several parts of the femoral component of the prosthesis (not present on previous films); periosteal reaction (medial and lateral aspects of femoral shaft).
(b) Infection or aseptic loosening of the prosthesis.
(c) A gallium[67] scan or CT scan; microscopy and culture of fluid aspirated from the hip (under ultrasound control).

The risks of sepsis in a hip joint prosthesis are greater in patients with RA compared to OA. Clinical presentation varies considerably according to the timing of the infection and the causative organism. Acute perioperative septic arthritis generally occurs within a few weeks of surgery and presents classical features of a swollen, painful warm joint, often with fever and peripheral leucocytosis. Most infections probably introduced during surgery, however, have a less dramatic presentation within the first year; local swelling and fever may be minimal or absent, and the diagnosis is suspected because of unexplained joint pain or inadequate function. The usual organism is Staphylococcus epidermidis, less commonly S. aureus, gram-negative bacilli, streptococci or anaerobes; mixed infections are not uncommon. Haematogenously acquired infections usually occur a year or more after surgery and have a subacute or chronic presentation. S. aureus and S. epidermidis are the usual organisms, settling around the prosthesis after a transient bacteremia, sometimes triggered by dental or other procedures (requirement for prophylactic antibiotics during dental and operative procedures is still debatable).
Chronic presentation of sepsis is very difficult to distinguish from mechanical aseptic loosening of the prosthesis. Pain only on weight-bearing is more consistent with aseptic loosening; pain is continuous with most infected prostheses. Radiographs may demonstrate radiolucencies and position change with subsidence or periosteal reaction. However, these changes occur late (three to six months of sepsis) and are also seen with mechanical loosening. Enhanced uptake on technetium diphosphonate bone scan at the bone-cement interface is normal for up to nine months post-arthroplasty; without serial scans for comparison it is only after nine to 12 months that increased activity is indicative of sepsis and/or loosening. Although focal increased uptake at one or more points around the prosthesis favours an inflammatory problem the scan cannot differentiate infection and loosening and therefore further investigations are necessary. A positive gallium[67] scan is strong indirect evidence of sepsis, and CT scanning is often useful in distinguishing the two conditions. Arthrography and aspiration are often diag-

nostic in the septic prosthetic hip; if needle aspiration is technically unsuccessful an open surgical procedure is warranted. Multiple specimens of synovial fluid and/or synovium/tissue should be cultured since organisms are often fastidious or may be mistaken for a contaminant.

Treatment of infected prostheses usually requires removal and surgical debridement as well as parenteral antibiotics; only 20–40% of infected prostheses are salvaged by drainage and prolonged antibiotics. In cases of mechanical loosening revision surgery can be delayed if symptoms are mild; occasional rapid bone resorption may make delayed surgery technically difficult. In this patient aspiration of synovial fluid under ultrasound control confirmed S. epidermidis infection. She underwent prosthesis reimplantation in a single procedure (using antibiotic-impregnated cement) though more commonly this is a two-stage procedure.

90 (a) Gross, asymmetric soft tissue swelling; changes of osteoarthritis (cartilage loss, subchondral erosion, osteophyte, lateral deviation) in multiple interphalangeal joints; cartilage loss in left midcarpal joint.
(b) Diuretic-induced (secondary) gout and pre-existing nodal OA.
(c) Attempt to stop diuretic. If impractical, prescribe low dose (100mg daily) allopurinol and monitor renal function and serum uric acid. Cautiously increase allopurinol to maintain uric acid levels in lower half of normal range.

In contrast to primary gout, diuretic-induced gout shows:
• later onset (seventh to ninth decades)
• reversed sex ratio (women more than men)
• presentation with tophi and chronic symptoms more than acute attacks
• early involvement of upper limbs
• frequent concurrence with nodal OA
• common association with impaired renal function
• common association with hypertension, cardiac failure (hence diuretic therapy)

This woman is typical in presenting with discharging tophi and exacerbation of her previously quiescent nodal OA. Discharging tophi associate with erythema and local inflammation and "infected Heberden's node" is invariably misdiagnosed. Monosodium urate monohydrate (MSUM) crystals macroscopically appear white and subcutaneous accumulations are often visibly pale; acutely inflamed tophi attract polymorphonuclear cells and give a yellow pus appearance.

Tissue changes that accompany osteoarthritis appear to enhance nucleation and growth of crystals, associating particularly with calcium pyrophosphate and apatite crystal deposition. The presence of such non-specific tissue factors (or absence of natural inhibitors) may explain the predilection of MSUM crystals to deposit in osteoarthritic hands. MSUM crystal deposition is slow, and it usually takes several years of diuretic therapy and hyperuricaemia to produce gout.

The radiograph of this patient shows osteoarthritis changes in a typical distribution. There are no specific radiographic features of gout, but features that suggest superadded gout are the asymmetric soft tissue swelling, the marked midcarpal chondropathy and the severity of interphalangeal joint damage.

Management of secondary gout in the elderly can prove problematic. Sometimes the diuretic can be stopped or substituted with an alternative antihypertensive agent with no hyperuricaemic effect. Otherwise hypouricaemic therapy is required. Most patients have mild to moderate renal impairment making allopurinol the appropriate drug (uricosurics are contraindicated with renal impairment). Unfortunately allopurinol toxicity is more frequent in the elderly, especially in those with renal impairment, so low doses (50–100mg daily) should be given initially and only increased slowly as required. Colchicine, as prophylaxis or treatment of acute attacks, should also be used with caution in low doses in the elderly, especially if there is renal impairment. NSAIDs are usually contra-indicated in such patients due to cardiac decompensation and gut toxicity, and simple analgesics are the mainstay for symptomatic control. Local steroid injections are reserved for acute attacks.

91 (a) Fusion of sacroiliac joints; calcification of anterior longitudinal ligament; marginal syndesmophytes; concentric joint space loss of hips; probable osteopenia.
(b) Ankylosing spondylitis (AS).
(c) Hips, knees, shoulders (though any joint may be involved).

Up to 20% of patients (particularly teenagers) present with peripheral arthropathy, usually asymmetric and involving large lower limb joints. Peripheral arthropathy can develop after the spinal disease has become inactive. At the hip concentric cartilage loss is characteristic; osteophyte response is usually "whiskery" and fibrous and bony ankylosis may develop.
Extra-articular manifestations of AS include general symptoms (fatigue, weight loss, low-grade fever) often with anaemia and a variable (usually modest) acute phase response (elevated ESR, viscosity, CRP). Iritis occurs in up to 25% of patients; this is unrelated to severity of the spondylitis but may associate with peripheral joint involvement. Iritis may affect both eyes but attacks are usually unilateral; episodes are often self-limiting but may require local or systemic steroids. Other manifestations rarely produce clinical problems but include:
• aortic incompetence, cardiomegaly, conduction defects
• upper lobe pulmonary fibrosis (classically left), sometimes complicated by cavitation and aspergillosis
• asymptomatic prostatitis (80% of men)
• amyloidosis
• cauda equina syndrome
Inflammatory bowel disease (Crohn's, ulcerative colitis) is a disease association rather than an extra-articular feature.
Syndesmophytes arise by inflammation, calcification and ossification of annulus fibrosus fibres. This initially erosive enthesopathy usually starts at the anterior vertebral corners ("Romanus lesion") which with associated periostitis of the anterior vertebral body leads to vertebral "squaring" with loss of anterior concavity; subsequent sclerosis of the Romanus lesion causes "shiny corners". New bone slowly replaces the annulus leading to vertical bridging syndesmophytes (with no/little loss of intervertebral space), and eventually to the classical "bamboo" spine. Accompanying apophyseal joint inflammation and eventual ankylosis further contribute to complete immo-

bility of the spine. Calcification of other fibrous structures, including the anterior longitudinal ligament, is a common late feature. In classic AS (and AS accompanying inflammatory bowel disease) syndesmophytes are typically symmetrical, fine and "marginal" (following the annulus fibres). Syndesmophytes in spondylitis of chronic Reiter's or psoriasis are more commonly asymmetrical, coarse and "non-marginal" (occurring outside the annulus and involving more of the vertebral body). Osteophytes mainly develop in the outer fibres of the annulus and are asymmetrical, growing out laterally rather than vertically, and often associating with intervertebral narrowing (ankylosis is not a feature). Ossification associated with DISH (Q. & A. 57) is coarse and attaches near the waist of the vertebra, often leaving a gap between the bridging bone and the anterior vertebral corners.

92 (a) Diabetic cheiroarthropathy ("stiff hands").
(b) Flexor tenosynovitis; bilateral Dupuytren's contractures; scleroderma.

Cheiroarthropathy is more common in non-insulin (75%) than insulin (30–50%) dependent diabetics, with positive correlations with disease duration and presence of renal or retinal microvascular disease. Flexion contractures result from increased dermal collagen which causes thickening and induration of skin and connective tissue (including capsule) particularly around MCPJs and PIPJs. The mechanism may relate to stabilisation of collagen from glycosylation of cross-links; similar collagen increase occurs in other tissues (eg lungs). Unlike skin thickening in scleroderma there is no finger pulp loss, altered pigmentation, Raynaud's or loss of skin appendages. Pain is not usually a feature and functional disturbance is the principal problem. Differentiation is principally from flexor tenosynovitis (+/- "trigger finger") and Dupuytren's contracture, both of which are more common in diabetics. Other musculoskeletal conditions increased in frequency in diabetes include:
• calcific periarthritis/bursitis
• adhesive capsulitis ("frozen shoulder"), which may sequentially affect both sides
• reflex sympathetic dystrophy (in neuropathic limbs)
• carpal tunnel syndrome
• osteomylitis
• Charcot joint (particularly tarsus, ankle)
• diffuse idiopathic skeletal hyperostosis (DISH), particularly in non-insulin dependent obese diabetics (possibly relating to increased insulin levels).

93 (a) Reflex sympathetic dystrophy syndrome (RSDS).
(b) Plain radiographs show diffuse regional osteopenia in established cases.

A bone scan will show diffuse increased uptake, being positive before radiographic osteopenia develops.
Thermography and skin potential measurements can demonstrate the vasomotor changes but are not widely available.
  RSDS (algodystrophy/painful regional osteoporosis) is an uncommon condition known by a variety of names. It occurs at any age, mainly in women. It may be idiopathic or follow an obvious triggering event (eg trau-

ma, neurological injury, ischaemic heart disease). Partial forms may be common though easily missed.

RSDS most commonly affects a whole hand or foot. The initial **acute phase** is characterised by pain, often severe and "burning", and extreme tenderness, hyperaesthesia and allodynia (discomfort resulting from usually non-painful stimuli such as light pressure) which restrict normal usage. Pitting/non-pitting oedema and vasomotor disturbance reflecting autonomic dysfunction (Raynaud's, vasodilatation, vasoconstriction, altered sweating) are usually present. After weeks or months pain and swelling subside as trophic skin changes develop (**dystrophic stage**). After further months subcutaneous atrophy and flexion contractures may develop (**atrophic stage**). The course is variable and early treatment may prevent subsequent atrophy.

The diagnosis is made clinically and supported by regional patchy osteopenia (or in early cases by positive bone scan) with absent acute phase response or hypercalcaemia. Arthropathy, including infection, is the principal differential diagnosis prior to investigation. In this patient RSDS was suggested by the severity and persistence of the pain which was out of proportion to the preceding injury. Management centres on early mobilisation to minimise and desensitize the abnormal autonomic reflex. A variety of interventions in addition to analgesics have been used to reduce pain and aid mobilisation, including vasoactive drugs (nifedipine, propanolol, phenoxybenzamine); corticosteroids; transcutaneous nerve stimulation; regional anaesthetic infusions; calcitonin; and chemical sympathetic blockade. Surgical sympathectomy is not generally advised. The earlier the treatment the more likely it is to be effective. Although usually self-limiting, some cases may persist for years.

94 (a) Fusiform swelling of middle and index PIPJs with loss of depth of overlying skin furrows; synovitis of second/third MCPJs producing swelling proximal to the joint line either side of the metacarpal head.
(b) Loss of distinct cortical outline either side of the metacarpal head (early non-proliferative marginal erosions); possible uniform joint space loss and juxta-articular osteopenia. These findings are typical of RA.

In RA proliferating synovial tissue produces marginal erosions at intra-articular sites unprotected by overlying cartilage ("bare" areas). Initial indistinctness of the cortical line ("dot-dash" or "brush-stroke" appearance) is followed by irregularity of bone contour; unlike seronegative spondarthropathy there is little accompanying bone proliferation. Cartilage loss, causing joint space narrowing, usually occurs later; it is diffuse and tends to affect all compartments of complex joints such as the wrist or knee (cf focal loss characteristic of OA, and generally preserved joint space characteristic of gout). Other radiographic features include:
• soft-tissue swelling (synovitis, bursae, tenosynovitis, tendinitis, nodules).
• osteopenia – juxta-articular (early) or generalised (late).
• osseous cysts ("geodes") – multiple, small subchondral lucencies that are occasionally large and extensive (especially in the hands of physically active men – "typus robustus").
• pressure erosions – extra-articular osseous defects arising from mass pressure effects from nodules, bursitis etc.

- compressive erosions – marked cartilage and bone attrition may permit one bone to compress and deform another (usually in joints exposed to forcible impact loading, eg protrusio at the hip, concertina deformities, or "arthritis mutilans" at small finger joints.
- deformity/subluxation (late) – characteristic for RA at individual sites, resulting from tendon, capsule, or ligament weakening/rupture as well as cartilage/bone attrition.
- spontaneous bony ankylosis – ocasionally wrist and midfoot (rare at other sites).
- stress fracture – particularly lower fibula or tibia (late, usually with osteopenia), or collapse of large osseous cysts.

Although joint involvement may be asymmetric in early disease, with unilateral neurologic deficits, or as a result of abnormal mechanical overusage, symmetry is an important and usual characteristic.

95 (a) Figure *a*: loss of lumbar lordosis; exaggerated smooth dorsal kyphosis; protuded neck; possible mild hip flexion. Figure *b*: virtually absent lumbar spine flexion; reduced hip flexion (the site where most anterior flexion is occurring).
(b) Ankylosing spondylitis (AS).

Despite chronic discomfort the majority of AS patients have a good prognosis with respect to maintaining a normal work and social lifestyle, only a few progressing to severe total ankylosis and major functional impairment. Regular exercise and attention to posture are the key aspects to management and depend on patient education and motivation. Swimming is the best routine sport; a firm mattress is better than a soft bed; regular extension exercises should become a daily routine; intermittent NSAIDs, analgesics and hot showers facilitate exercises during phases of symptom exacerbation. Intermittent physiotherapy, hydrotherapy and remedial exercise may benefit resistant cases. Second-line agents such as sulphasalazine are helpful for peripheral joint involvement and may reduce axial inflammation (this is harder to assess). Hip replacement is required for severe arthropathy; surgical correction of advanced spinal flexion is reserved for specialist units.

It is important to serially monitor for slow, often imperceptible, functional decline that justifies more aggressive management. Spinal movements symetrically decrease in AS (cf. mechanical back problems) and a number of spinal measurements may be used, including:
- Schober test: a mark is made 5cm below and 10cm above a line joining the dimples of Venus and the distance remeasured after full anterior flexion (distraction of >5 cm is expected in normals).
- chest expansion (measured through nipple-line; costovertebral involvement, normally >5cm).
- finger-to-floor distance (Figure *b*: combined spine and hip movement).
- occiput-to-wall distance (patient standing upright, heels back against wall, eyes level, indicating cervical/thoracic spine fixed flexion).
- intermalleolar straddle: the distance between medial malleoli during maximum bilateral hip abduction (indicating overall pelvic mobility and enthesopathy).

96 (a) Supraspinatus tendon lesion; subacromial bursitis.
(b) A supraspinatus lesion (tendinitis or mild tear).

Lesions of the rotator cuff, particularly the supraspinatus portion close to its humeral head insertion, are very common and range from mild tendinitis in a young patient to a complete tear in an older patient. Typical features in the history include:
• defined onset of pain in a single region
• often follows strenuous or unaccustomed exercise
• pain limited to only one or a few movements of the shoulder
• non-progressive symptoms
   Adhesive capsulitis ("frozen shoulder") often has a defined onset but pain initially progresses and then resolves as stiffness and limited mobility become dominant. Glenohumeral arthropathy occurs mainly in the setting of multiple regional pain and shows variable progression; eventually most movements may be painful. Rotator cuff lesions and glenohumeral arthropathy both cause referred pain maximal in the upper outer aspect of the arm.
   "Hands behind head" is a useful screen for shoulder problems. It involves glenohumeral abduction and external rotation (the two movements first and most severely affected by arthropathy) and utilises (lightly stresses) the muscles/tendons of the posterior rotator cuff.
   A painful middle arc may occur with supraspinatus tendon lesions or subacromial bursitis (both get compressed as the humeral head rises against the coracoacromial arch in mid elevation). If this man had isolated subacromial bursitis resisted active abduction (Figure *b*) would not have been painful; pain reproduced by this manoeuvre supports a supraspinatus tendon lesion (his retained strength is against a major tear). Resisted active external rotation (infraspinatus/teres minor) and internal rotation (subscapularis) complete the testing of the cuff.
   Absence of anterior glenohumeral joint-line/capsular tenderness and crepitus with full, pain-free passive external rotation (Figure *c*) excludes synovitis or capsulitis. This manoeuvre provides a useful "minimal" assessment of the glenohumeral joint. This man responded symptomatically to an NSAID and ultrasound therapy and did not require local injection of steroid. He was also given a strengthening programme of exercises under initial physiotherapy supervision.

97 (a) Features of OA, namely joint space narrowing (MCPJs, IPJs, first CMCJ); osteophyte (DIPJs); sclerosis (DIPJs, first CMCJ); lateral deviation (DIPJs). Synovial/capsular calcification and soft tissue swelling (MCPJs). Chondrocalcinosis of triangular ligament.
(b) Chronic pyrophosphate arthropathy (CPA).

CPA predominates in elderly women and is characterised by calcium pyrophosphate dihydrate (CPPD) crystal deposition and structural changes showing radiographic features of OA. Features which may distinguish CPA from OA include:
• florid inflammatory component (stiffness, large effusions)
• accompanying hand tenosynovitis (uncommon)
• superimposition of acute attacks ("pseudogout")

136

- frequent involvement of two or three knee compartments (often mainly patellofemoral) with subsequent valgus as well as varus deformities (a) (OA mainly results in varus deformity)
- atypical distribution (radiocarpal, glenohumeral, elbow and ankle joints are commonly affected in CPA, uncommonly in OA)
- CPPD crystals in synovial fluid
- radiographic chondrocalcinosis
- calcification of synovium/capsule (uncommonly tendons, bursae)
- "hypertrophic" radiographic features with predominance of osteophyte and cysts
- occasional severe destructive change

In some patients the combination of overt synovitis and atypical joint distribution may suggest RA, particularly if accompanied by periarticular complications such as carpal tunnel syndrome or tenosynovitis ("pseudorheumatoid" presentation). Modest elevation of ESR in CPA, and weakly positive rheumatoid factor in the elderly, are both common and may cause further confusion. On the other hand, Heberden's nodes (Figure *b*) are common in the elderly and their presence would not mitigate against the diagnosis of superimposed RA.

The helpful investigations in this situation are (a) synovial fluid analysis to confirm CPPD crystals, (b) plain radiographs to show features of CPA (Figure *c*) but no marginal erosions, osteopenia or widespread chondropathy of RA.

Although RA negatively associates with CPPD crystal deposition the two conditions occasionally coexist (by comparison coexistent RA and gout is extremely rare). In coexistent disease radiographic features of RA may be modified and appear atypical with respect to:
- retained bone density
- paucity of erosions
- prominent osteophyte and remodelling
- prominent cysts

This woman had no extra-articular features (eg nodules, scleritis), only a modest acute phase response, and no marginal erosions on radiographs (hands, feet, shoulders, knees). Aspiration of her knees confirmed CPPD. Her clinical features and investigations were therefore consistent with a diagnosis of CPA alone.

98 (a) Livedo reticularis.
(b) SLE.
(c) Mild or moderate anaemia (normochromic, normocytic); leucopenia (particularly lymphopaenia); moderate or severe thrombocytopoenia. Cytotoxic therapy may result in decreased blood elements and macrocytosis (azathioprine).

SLE-specific skin lesions include the acute butterfly rash, subacute cutaneous LE (SCLE), and discoid lupus. SLE-nonspecific lesions include mucosal ulceration, panniculitis, alopecia, vasculitis and livedo reticularis. Livedo is common in normal subjects, especially women; it mainly affects the inside leg and forearm and is worsened by cold. More widespread livedo is suggestive of an underlying connective tissue problem. The combination of Raynaud's, arthralgia, photosensitivity and livedo in a woman strongly suggests lupus. An association between livedo and cerebrovascular accident (Sneddon's syndrome) was subsequently expanded to include vascular thrombosis (arterial/venous), thrombocytopenia, pregnancy loss and persistently elevated levels of antiphospholipid antibodies (antiphospholipid syndrome); other features, such as migraine, have also been added. This syndrome may coexist with SLE.

Blood elements may be low in SLE due to reduced production and/or increased consumption. Haemolytic anaemia may associate with splenomegaly, cold agglutinins and a positive direct Coomb's test. Antibodies against platelets and leucocytes also occur.

The ESR is usually raised in active SLE; CRP is usually normal or only modestly raised (if very high consider superimposed infection). Hypergammaglobulinaemia is common, cryoglobulinaemia uncommon. About a third of patients are seropositive for rheumatoid factor (rarely high titre). Useful immunological tests include:
- serum complement (C_3, C_4); low levels reflect disease activity, very low levels suggest renal involvement (rarely congenital deficiency). Since these proteins are acute phase reactants an increase in their degradation products (eg C_3dg) is a better guide to activation.
- antinuclear antibodies (ANA); this has very high sensitivity (ANA-negative SLE is very rare), but poor specificity, for SLE (high titres increase disease specificity). Other associations with ANA include other major connective tissue diseases (RA, scleroderma, polymyositis, Sjögrens), myasthenia gravis, chronic active hepatitis, juvenile chronic arthritis, and thyroiditis. Normal subjects may be ANA-positive.

Various types of ANA may be identified according to immunofluorescent staining pattern or specific substrate. For example:
- Anti double-stranded DNA antibody – highly specific, but relatively insensitive, for SLE; titres correlate with disease activity.
- ENA (extractable nuclear antigen) antibodies. These include:
  Anti-RNP (ribonucleoprotein); common in SLE, MCTD
  Anti-Sm (10–30%); high specificity for SLE
  Anti-Ro (SS-A); associated with ANA-negative lupus, neonatal lupus, SCLE
  Anti-La (SS-B); associated with Sjögrens, SLE

99 (a) Extensive regional osteopenia (proximal femur, much of hemipelvis).
(b) Transient osteoporosis of the hip (TOH).
(c) Pregnant women (third trimester, immediately post-partum).

TOH is considered a form of algodystrophy though its aetiology is speculative. Peripheral autonomic dysfunction has been suggested, possibly caused in late pregnancy by pressure on the obturator nerve, ischaemia or hormonal alterations. It mainly affects healthy middle-aged men but pregnant women are also particularly affected (children rarely). The left hip is involved more often than the right; recurrence and bilateral (but not synchronous) involvement are reported. Three distinctive phases are described:
1. Progressive pain and functional disability (first month).
2. Appearance of radiographic osteopenia around time of maximum symptoms (second to third month).
3. Symptom regression and gradual remineralisation to normal (c.six to nine months).

Established radiographic changes are characteristic. Osteopenia is regional and often dramatic; in severe cases the bone architecture in parts is difficult to see. Importantly, joint space is invariably preserved. Bone scans are positive before radiographic osteopenia and confirm the regional nature of the condition at an early stage (homogeneous uptake centering on the femoral head is typical). A CT scan will confirm joint space integrity and local demineralisation and exclude alternative pathology. MRI scans show transient marrow oedema with reduced T_1 and increased T_2 signal; these typical medullary signs help differentiation from bone tumour, osteomylitis and possible accompanying stress fracture. All blood investigations (including ESR, CRP, calcium, cultures) are normal. The clinical differential diagnosis may include inflammatory joint disease, septic arthritis (including TB), metastatic disease, multiple myeloma, pigmented villonodular synovitis, stress fracture and osteonecrosis; screening blood tests and plain x-ray (with or without bone scan) usually permits a speedy diagnosis.

Treatment is restricted weight-bearing (to alleviate symptoms and prevent stress microfractures) with appropriate analgesia. NSAIDs, oral and intra-articular steroids, sympathetic blocks, hydrotherapy, and traction do not appear to alter the course of TOH, though calcitonin may hasten healing rates.

100 (a) Osteopenia; anterior vertebral wedging and decreased intervertebral space at several levels.
(b) Vertebral fractures.
(c) Idiopathic/post-menopausal osteoporosis.

Osteoporosis is characterised by low bone mass with increased risk of fracture (especially vertebral bodies, femoral neck, distal radius/ulna; less commonly proximal humerus, pelvis). Pain from fracture is the only symptom. The diagnosis is essentially by exclusion. This patient's screening tests suggested no underlying metabolic or malignant disease as a cause of osteopenia and vertebral fracture. Conditions to consider include:
• osteomalacia; not uncommon in elderly, especially Asians, and readily treatable; usually suggested by biochemistry though bone biopsy is defini tive investigation.
• malignancy (especially myeloma)
• Paget's disease
• hyperparathyroidism, hyperthyroidism
• osteomyelitis (unlikely to give recurrent self-limiting episodes)

The screening investigations undertaken in this woman usually suffice, though a bone scan and/or biopsy may be indicated in cases with atypical clinical features or radiographs.

Factors that predispose to idiopathic, post-menopausal osteoporosis include:
• ageing/gender; peak bone mass is reached in mid-thirties then declines c.1% per year.
• menopause (natural or following oophorectomy): a major association, diminished oestrogen and progestogen levels resulting in accelerated bone loss (c.3–5% per year for c.10 years)
• genetics/race; there is an increased susceptibility in certain populations, particularly if they have low peak bone mass and lean/small body mass.

Prevalence order is whites > Asians > blacks. Unidentified factors appear to operate in some families (with high concordance in monozygotic twins and mothers/daughters).
- reduced mobility, low levels of physical activity.
- smoking, excessive alcohol (especially in men).
- drugs: glucocorticoids, prolonged heparin (possibly NSAIDs).

Acute vertebral crush fractures are managed by: (a) **pain relief**, using appropriate combinations of simple analgesics, NSAIDs, opiates, anxiolytic/psychotropics, and (b) **initial rest** (one to two days) followed by **early mobilisation** to prevent detrimental spinal muscle weakness and enhanced bone loss. Measures to slow down further bone loss and to reduce fracture incidence should be considered in those at high risk or following presentation with fracture. Suggested useful measures include;
- regular exercise; several hours each week of walking and gentle training that involves impact loading
- dietary advice (ensuring adequate vitamin D intake and sunlight expo sure) and possible calcium supplementation (c.800mg/day)
- reduction/cessation of smoking and alcohol
- hormone replacement therapy (for five years) for women within ten years of menopause (warn patient of possible cyclical mastalgia and menstrua tion)
- cyclical etidronate (for three years); this diphonsphonate inhibits osteoclast activity; it is given in 12-week cycles (two weeks – etidronate 400mg/day; ten weeks – calcium).

INDEX

143